Drug Design - Novel Advances in the Omics Field and Applications

Edited by Arli Aditya Parikesit

Published in London, United Kingdom

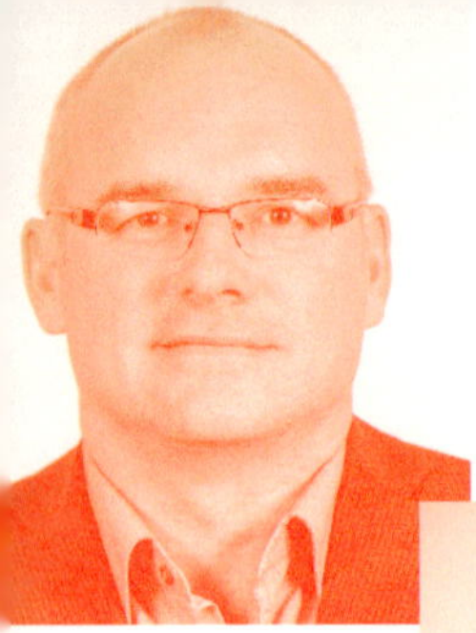
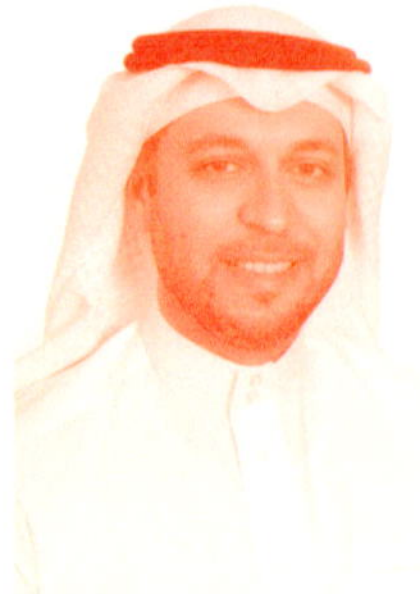
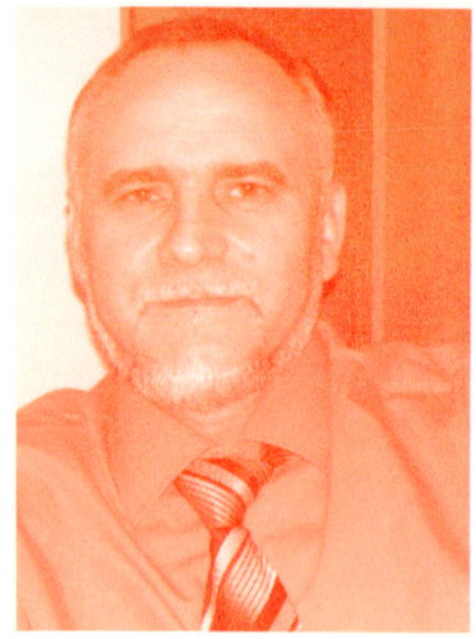
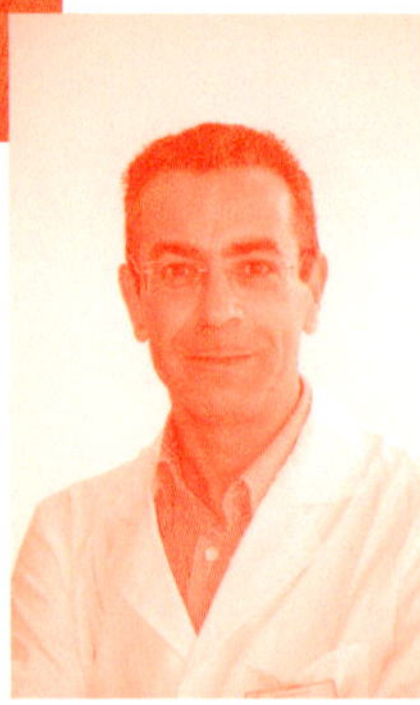
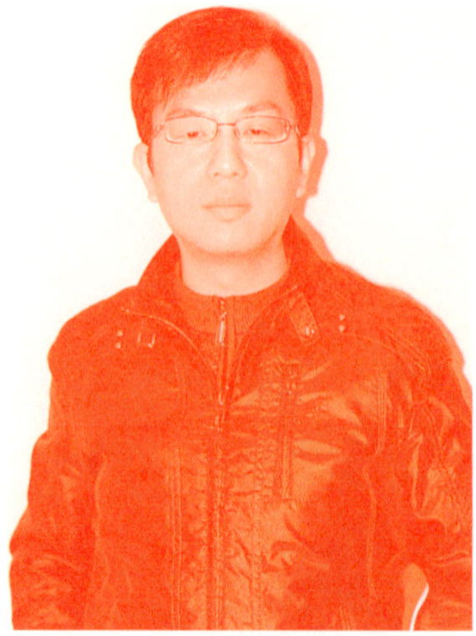
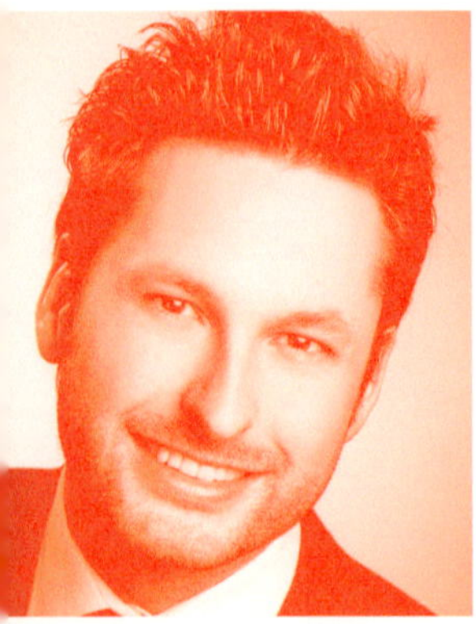
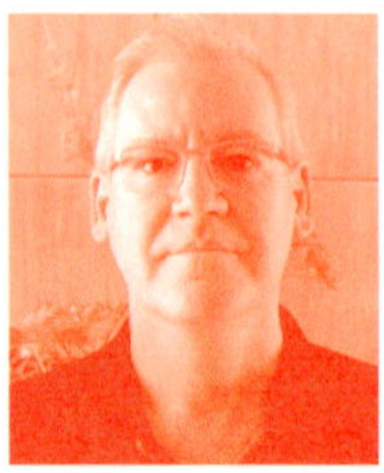

IntechOpen

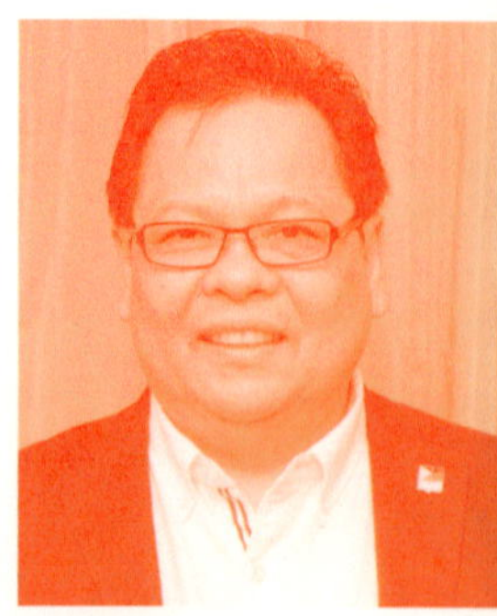
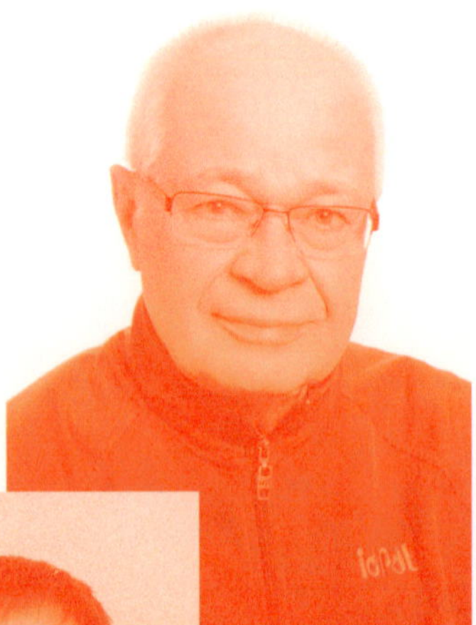
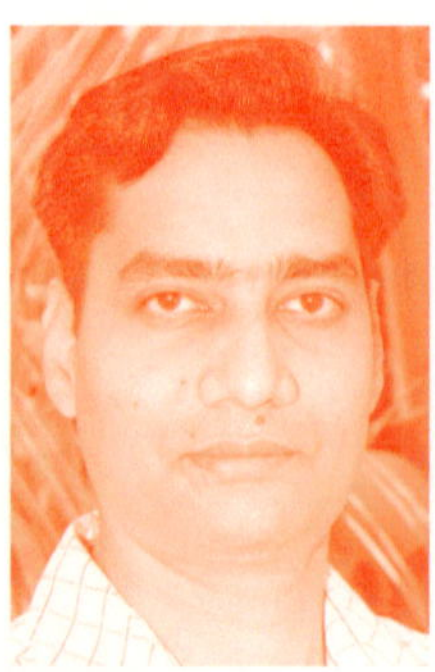
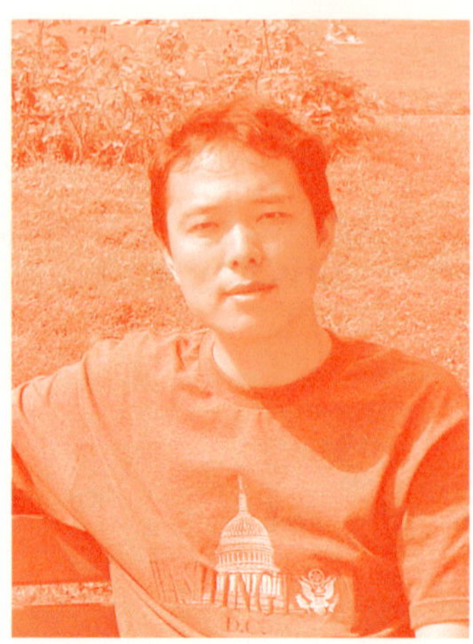
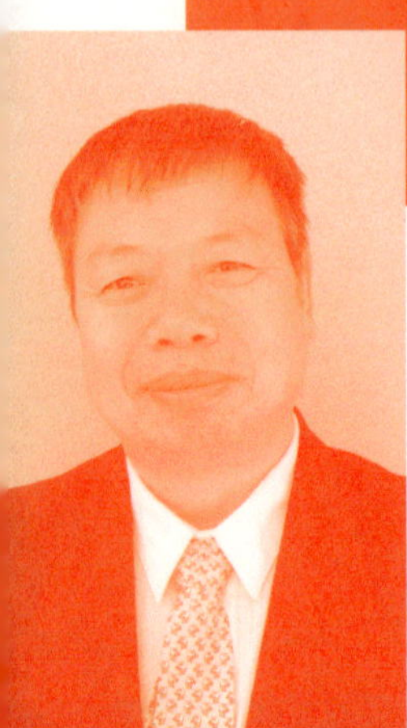
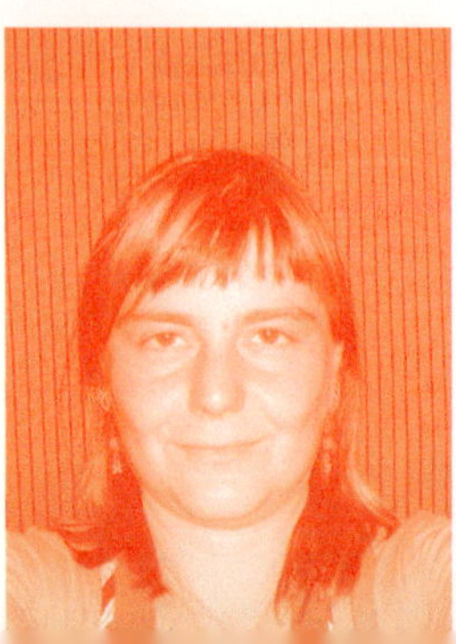

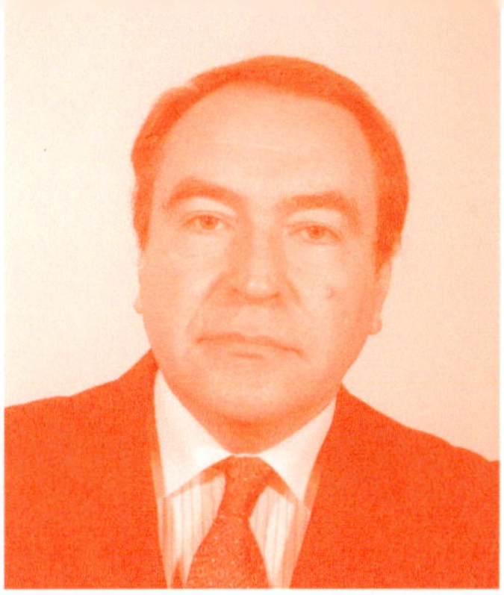
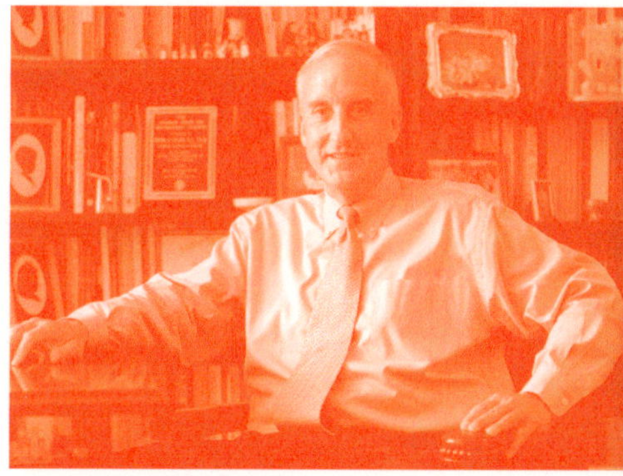
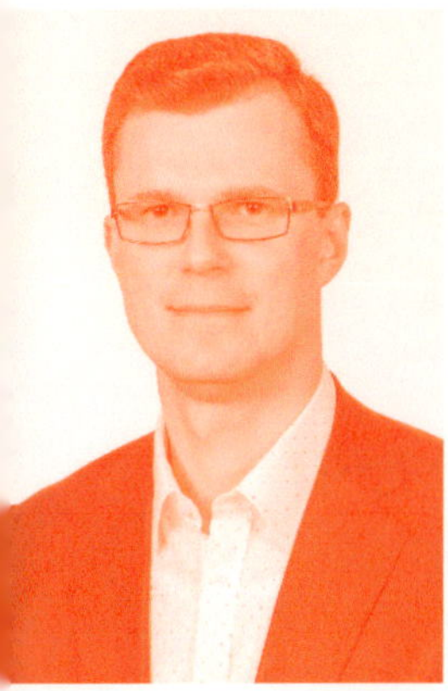
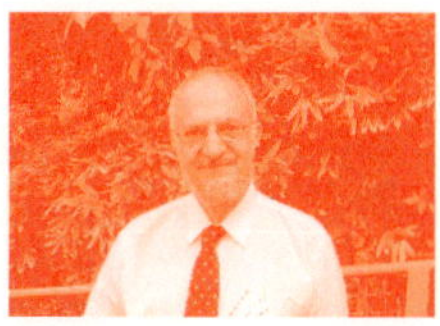
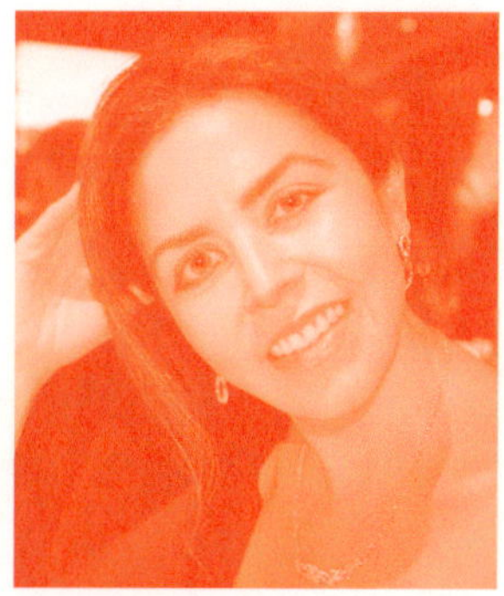

Supporting open minds since 2005

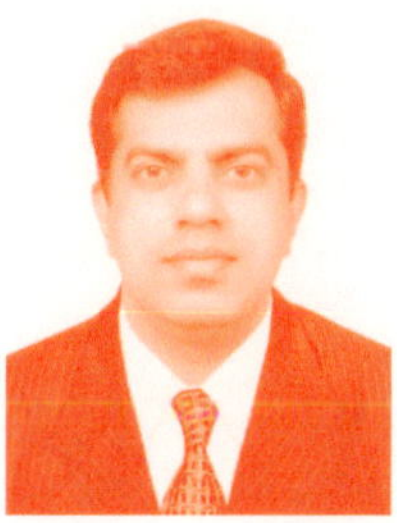
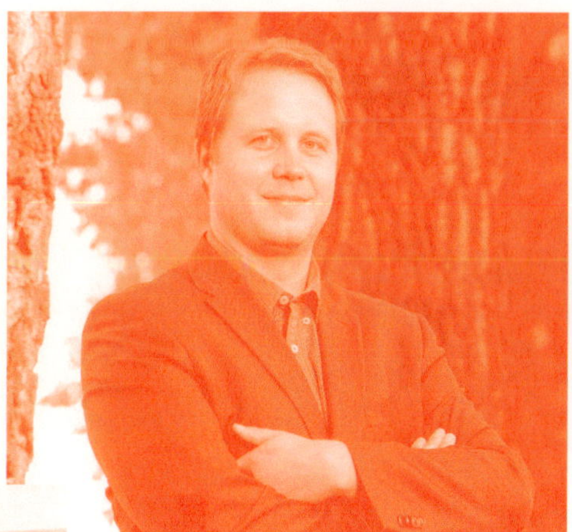
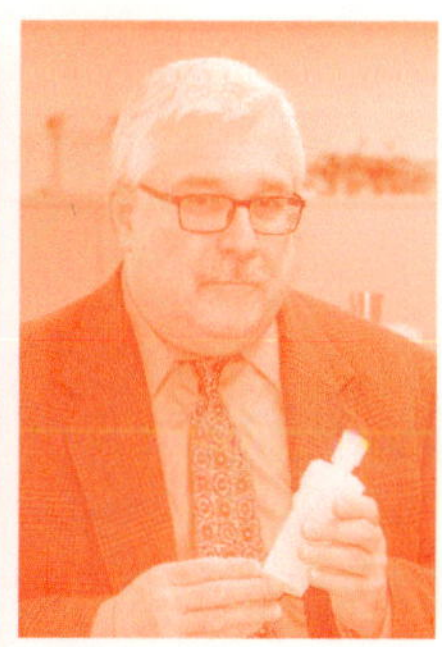
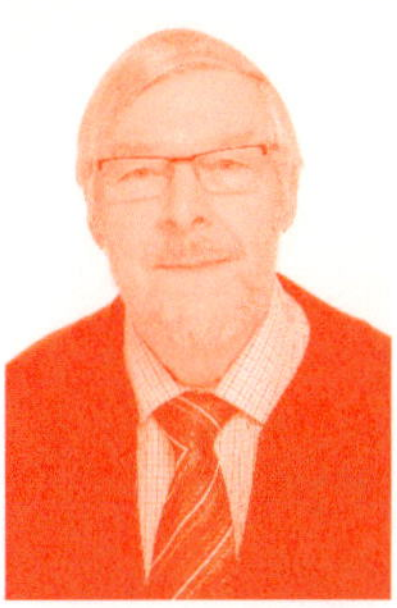
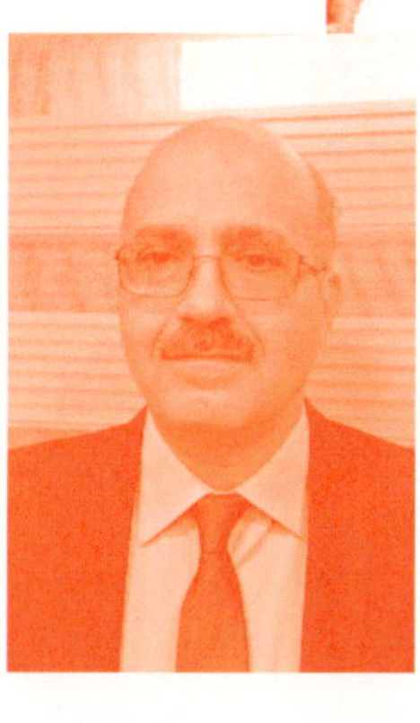
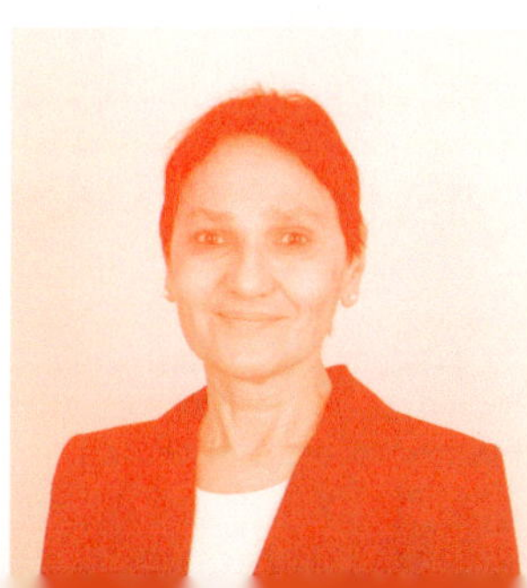
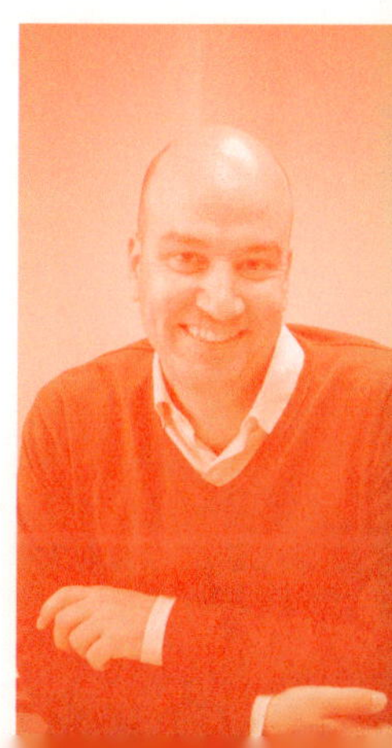

Drug Design - Novel Advances in the Omics Field and Applications
http://dx.doi.org/10.5772/intechopen.87640
Edited by Arli Aditya Parikesit

Contributors
Brindha Devi Parthiban, Thanga Ridhanya, Rahul Shukla, Abdul Hameed Khan, Maria Elizbeth Alvarez Sanchez, Julio C. Torres-Romero, Julio César Lara-Riegos, Sushally Uc-Colli, Edgar Antonio Estrella-Parra, Victor Arana-Argaez, Veronica Fernandez-Sanchez, Mario Alberto Ramirez Camacho, Miguel Angel Peña Rico, Maria Dolores Ponce Regalado, Safna Hussan Kodakkat Parambil, Ioana Berindan-Neagoe, Laura-Ancuta Pop, Oana Zanoaga, Paul Chiroi, Andreea Nutu, Cristina Stefan, Alexandru Irimie, Schuyler S. Korban, Arli Aditya Parikesit, Indulekha Jayarajan Jithin Raj, Sailaja Urpayil, Mohamed Shahin Thayyil

First published in London, United Kingdom, 2021 by IntechOpen
IntechOpen is the global imprint of INTECHOPEN LIMITED, registered in England and Wales, registration number: 11086078, 5 Princes Gate Court, London, SW7 2QJ, United Kingdom
Printed in Croatia

British Library Cataloguing-in-Publication Data
A catalogue record for this book is available from the British Library

Additional hard and PDF copies can be obtained from orders@intechopen.com

Drug Design - Novel Advances in the Omics Field and Applications
Edited by Arli Aditya Parikesit
p. cm.
Print ISBN 978-1-78984-752-9
Online ISBN 978-1-78984-753-6
eBook (PDF) ISBN 978-1-78985-201-1

For EU product safety concerns:
IN TECH d.o.o., Prolaz Marije Krucifikse Kozulić 3, 51000 Rijeka, Croatia, info@intechopen.com or visit our website at intechopen.com.

Meet the editor

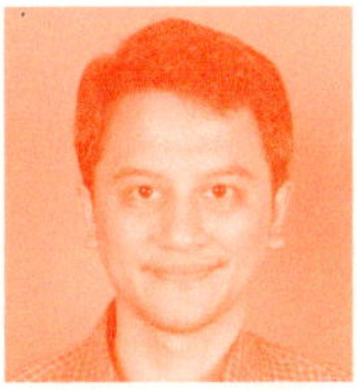

Dr. rer. nat. Arli Aditya Parikesit is the head of the Bioinformatics Department at Indonesia International Institute for Life Sciences (I3L). He finished both his bachelor's and master's degrees in chemistry at the Faculty of Mathematics and Natural Sciences, University of Indonesia. In order to pursue a degree in Bioinformatics, he accepted an offer from DAAD (German Academic Exchange Service) to conduct doctorate research at the Bioinformatics Group, Faculty of Informatics and Mathematics, University of Leipzig, Germany. His doctoral research is focused on the utilization of modern protein domain annotation techniques to the three domains of life. In addition, Dr. Arli is also an expert on immunoinformatics, bioinformatics algorithm, structural bioinformatics, in silico drug design, and in silico transcriptomics. Currently, Dr. Arli is devising a pipeline to apply his expertise to COVID-19 drug and vaccine designs.

Contents

Preface

The life sciences domain has entered a new paradigm shift when the World Health Organization (WHO) announced the COVID-19 pandemic in March 2020. In this regard, bioscientists worldwide were forced to accelerate their research efforts to a new level, as the world is desperately waiting for the development of the drug and vaccine to deter the SARS-CoV-2 virus. Up to this day, we have observed more than 3.3 million mortalities worldwide, and in many countries, their public health systems have been under the extra burden with almost all of their ICU beds occupied. However, as we learn that many health-related problems, such as malnutrition, could be resolved with advances in life sciences, such as the development of bioinformatics and nutrigenomics, we have a high hope that the latest breakthrough in this area could also assist us against this pandemic. Luckily, there are hopes in the air.

Right before the COVID-19 pandemic declared by the WHO, life sciences have incited novel areas of studies that revolutionize the health sector. They are the studies of structural bioinformatics, pharmacogenomics, and metabolomics. The structural bioinformatics field is the very foundation of the drug design research, as it provides insight into the molecular simulations and interactions between the biomolecules and the drug candidates. Secondly, pharmacogenomics is the starting point of any efforts in developing personalized medicine. Lastly, metabolomics provides instrumentation to elicit biomarkers for various diseases and health conditions. These studies have enabled current accelerated effort in COVID-19 research, as well as other diseases.

This book is mainly divided into two sections. The first one, "Omics Studies in Drug Design", discusses with a focus on pharmacogenomics and parts of metabolomics studies, mainly lipoproteomics and probiogenomics. In the second one, "Rational Drug Design", structural bioinformatics, and pharmaceutical chemistry experts collaborate and provide their insight into various diseases such as cancer. Their contributions are paramount to the studies of life sciences and enable further progress for eradicating life-threatening diseases such as COVID-19 and cancer.

To this end, although the world is currently ravaged by the COVID-19 pandemic, other kinds of diseases still stay with us. The HIV/AIDS pandemic is not over yet; tuberculosis is threatening us with antibiotic-resistant strains; cardiovascular disease is still considered the primary course of mortality in many countries; and not to mention there are still other noncommunicable diseases such as cancer, diabetes, and neurological disorders. With so many challenges ahead of us, it is expected that the scientific breakthrough, as elicited in this book, will eventually shed light on how to eradicate, or at least tame, those maladies and provide hope to humanity.

Arli Aditya Parikesit
Head of Bioinformatics Department,
School of Life Sciences,
Indonesia International Institute for Life Sciences (I3L),
Indonesia

Section 1

Omics Studies in Drug Design

Chapter 1

Introductory Chapter: The Emerging Corner of the Omics Studies for Rational Drug Design

Arli Aditya Parikesit

1. Introduction

1.1 Structural bioinformatics contributions in -omics studies

The Acceleration of COVID-19 research in Proteomics and Transcriptomics studies occurred swiftly due to the massive amount of investment and advances in biomanufacturing [1, 2]. Moreover, the repurposing drug research has elicited remdesivir as the FDA-approved drug for COVID-19, despite mixed result from the WHO solidarity trial [3]. More drug leads are also currently undergoing clinical trial as well. This rapid development in the rational drug design is strongly associated with the field of structural bioinformatics. As for now (Early December 2020), there are more than 600 deposited SARS-CoV-2 Protein structures in the PDB (per December 2020, in the http://www.rcsb.org). They are SARS-CoV-2 Proteins with various conformations, and bindings with various ligands [4]. Hence, those proteins structures and their annotated functions are currently subject of the extensive COVID-19 drug development along with hefty investment from the pharmaceutical companies. However, in the other side of the story, non-protein biomolecular structures are currently still off the radar. There are only handful of initiatives for the COVID-19 transcriptomics-based drugs [5–7]. However, drug-based transcriptomics initiatives in canceromics are more mature. Breast cancer transcriptomics-based leads are currently under development [8–10]. That particular progress could be elicited due to the application of structural bioinformatics method for prediction the 2D and 3D model of the nucleic acids [11]. However, massive clinical applications still in favors for the proteomics-based drugs due to the stability of the bioassay experiments. In the area of natural products computation, the only realistic approach is still the proteomics-based one. For instance, propolis, as a resinous material from bees, was a subject of intensive molecular simulation research for its respective compounds constituency as diabetes drug candidates [12]. Hence, the same material also employed for the possibility as COVID-19 leads compound [13]. Moreover, various secondary metabolite sources were also investigated as drug candidates with the molecular simulation research, such as ayurvedic plants of India, and various sources of Chinese herbal medicine [14–18]. In this regard, bioinformaticians should proceed with mindful and prudent manner on the deployment of the molecular docking method as there are validation issues that should be resolved before working on the samples [19, 20]. That includes the utilization of the docking decoys, reiterations of Tc-PLIF value, cross-docking, redocking of the attached ligand, and the refinement of the RMSD parameter [21–25]. However, the easiest validation method is the ligand redocking, provided the structure is exist in the PDB repository. The decoy deployment is the most computationally extensive of all, albeit of its high accuracy [26]. In this end, the measurement of the computational cost should be taken into consideration when applying molecular simulation is needed [27].

2. Pharmacogenomics and personalized medicine

Although it is still in its infancy, currently there is research that investigates the tendency that certain population group will be more vulnerable to COVID-19. For instance, Population with gene pool of Neanderthals was predicted to be vulnerable considerably [28]. In Indonesia, pharmacogenomics study has elicited correlation between anti-tuberculosis drug-induced liver injury (AT-DILI) severity and NAT2 phenotypes [29]. Moreover, expression of Long non-coding RNA (lncRNA) in diabetic patient is a useful lead for the progression of the epigenetic repertoire in the human cell [30]. Then, Molecular genomic is playing important role to annotate the cardiac function analysis [31]. The 7-day regiment deployment of the malaria drug primaquine is tolerated for patient with normal level of glucose-6-phosphate dehydrogenase (G6PD). Moreover, the resistance tendency of certain population group against malaria parasite has been observed as well [32]. Cancer is one of the most extensively studied disease in the pharmacogenomics field, in the light of the intensive computational biology tools, as tendencies for prevalence were elucidated in different races [33, 34]. Thus, the progress of epigenetics research has leveraged the pharmacogenomics field with various findings of biomarkers for cancer [35]. The various progresses in the pharmacogenomics field have shown that the molecular mechanism of diseases is beginning to be uncovered accordingly, especially with the development of epigenetics marker database [36]. Bioinformatics also play important role in annotating pharmacogenomics data, especially for the development of the genomics database and the disease-outcome prediction methods [37].

3. Metabolomics and disease biomarkers

The forefront of the metabolomics research is mainly the standard instrument in the analytical biochemistry such as HPLC and GC–MS, and also some supporting organic chemistry instrumentation such as C-NMR, H-NMR, UV, and IR [28–30, 38–40]. However, the deployment of the data science approach in interpretation of the metabolomics data enables the analysis of the large data sets, and eventually the data annotation in the biological database [41, 42]. Natural products research is one of the most dynamic fronts in the metabolomics research. Herbal medicine clinical trial toward COVID-19 patients show acceptable result for patients with mild symptoms, provided that the standard therapy still apply [43–45]. Moreover, secondary metabolite could serve as disease biomarkers. Insulin-resistant individuals will have decreased serum level of glycine, and also poor biotin metabolism [46]. Currently, probiotic metabolites are undergone extensive research to determine their possible anti-SARS-CoV-2 properties [47]. Propolis studies are also focused on the metabolomics side in order to provide sufficient data to the structural bioinformatics research, especially to determine the inhibitory activities against the SARS-CoV-2 virus [48–51]. Up to today, there are still limited number of the approved natural product based drugs, such as aspirin, penicillin, and taxol [52]. Bioinformatics research has been optimized to develop a more comprehensive biological conclusion in natural product chemistry, such as the annotation of naringin role in cancer, bioactive compounds of *Zingeber officinale,* and caffeine-aspirin interaction [53–55]. So more efforts should be elicited to improve the completeness of the natural products library, mainly to supplement the standard chemical compounds library such as Pubchem, and drug database such as drugbank. Hence, biomarkers could be elicited not only as small organic molecules, but also as larger biomolecules. For instance, the insulin level is one of the indicator of the diabetes progression, and indicator for the therapeutic options available [56]. Diabetic biomarker could be manifested as non-coding RNA as well [57, 58].

4. Medicinal chemistry and drug design in omics study

The metabolomics study is definitely inseparable from medicinal chemistry due to their overlapping domain [59]. The development of the metabolomics library enables the construction of the rich chemical-structures library, as well as their respective functional groups from the natural products [57–62]. Custom-made library will supplement the existing libraries, such as the pubchem, drugbank, and KEGG database [63–65]. In this regard, the availability of the functional-groups library will support the fragment-based drug design, where specialized algorithm was devised to inhibit every corner of the protein's cavity [66, 67]. Hence, the main challenge of this approach will be in the medicinal chemistry perspective, when extrapolating the in silico research into the in vitro one become necessary. Synthesizing custom-made compounds from fragment library will not be straightforward due to the special reaction condition needed, the existence of the new structural backbone, and the availability of the chemical regents [68]. In this end, the current standing of the medicinal chemistry field is still depend upon the derivatization of the current structural library of compounds, in order to develop new lead with feasible reaction conditions [69]. Metabolomics plays dominant role in developing such library. One of the application of this particular approach is the development of ceftaroline, which is a fifth-generation broad-spectrum cephalosporin antibiotic [70].

5. Outlook

Parallelization in the Drug Biomanufacturing with incremental optimization will facilitate the pipeline of therapeutic agent development [71, 72]. Such biomanufacturing efforts will be enhanced with the implementation of Artificial Intelligence (AI) for massive drug screening that could be beneficial for multi-components drug lead such as herbal medication, and machine-learning based implementation for such pipelines has been devised accordingly in COVID-19 leads development [73–76]. The extensive utilization of the common data science methods in bioinformatics, such as machine learning, will eventually provide insight that the management of life sciences data requires more than just becoming application users [77]. Massive automation efforts in the field of life sciences will eventually push forward with the inevitable integration with formal sciences, namely with both computer science and data science [78]. In this end, Bioinformatics will play important role to manage the experimental data from the life sciences lab [79]. For instance, utilization of the SUPERFAMILY and Gene Ontology database for annotating the protein domain expression of the *Plasmodium sp.* parasite could be a doable venue [80, 81]. Thus, the promises that already delivered by the omics studies will eventually shed light to the current state of the COVID-19 pandemic (per December 2020), and could elicit various therapeutic options for many more infectious diseases. However, non-communicable disease such as various types of cancer and diabetes will remain a challenging task to resolve as they invoke deep understanding of the human immunological system. It involves the utilization of the immunoinformatics tools that proceed beyond this chapter [82, 83]. Hence, it should be reminded that the basic sciences behind the omics studies could not be overlooked. Medicinal chemistry, biochemistry, molecular biology, biomedicine and biotechnology will remain important, as well as emerging sciences such as bioinformatics and data sciences.

Acknowledgements

The authors would like to thank the Institute for Research and Community Services (LPPM) of Indonesia International Institute for Life Sciences (I3L) for their heartfelt support. Thanks also go to the Indonesian Society for Bioinformatics and Biodiversity (ISBB) or *Masyarakat Bioinformatika dan Biodiversitas Indonesia* (MABBI) members and leaders for the thorough forum group discussion on the topic of COVID-19 pandemic, artificial intelligence for drug design, and molecular docking validation.

Author details

Arli Aditya Parikesit
Department of Bioinformatics, School of Life Sciences, Indonesia International Institute for Life Sciences, Jl. Pulomas Barat Kav.88, Jakarta, 13210, Indonesia

*Address all correspondence to: arli.parikesit@i3l.ac.id

References

[1] J.H. Martin, N.A. Bowden, Drug repurposing in the era of COVID-19: a call for leadership and government investment, Med. J. Aust. 212 (2020) 450-452.e1. https://doi.org/10.5694/mja2.50603.

[2] D.J. Payne, L.F. Miller, D. Findlay, J. Anderson, L. Marks, Time for a change: addressing R&D and commercialization challenges for antibacterials, Philos. Trans. R. Soc. B Biol. Sci. 370 (2015) 20140086. https://doi.org/10.1098/rstb.2014.0086.

[3] M. Gadebusch Bondio, M. Marloth, The "Historic Study" SOLIDARITY—Research's Answer to the Sars-CoV-2 Pandemic, NTM Int. J. Hist. Ethics Nat. Sci. Technol. Med. (2020). https://doi.org/10.1007/s00048-020-00257-5.

[4] F.K. Yoshimoto, The Proteins of Severe Acute Respiratory Syndrome Coronavirus-2 (SARS CoV-2 or n-COV19), the Cause of COVID-19, Protein J. 39 (2020) 198-216. https://doi.org/10.1007/s10930-020-09901-4.

[5] A.A. Parikesit, R. Nurdiansyah, The Predicted Structure for the Anti-Sense siRNA of the RNA Polymerase Enzyme (RdRp) gene of the SARS-CoV-2, Ber. Biol. 19 (2020) 97-108. https://doi.org/10.14203/beritabiologi.v19i1.3849.

[6] H. Uludağ, K. Parent, H.M. Aliabadi, A. Haddadi, Prospects for RNAi Therapy of COVID-19, Front. Bioeng. Biotechnol. (2020). https://doi.org/10.3389/fbioe.2020.00916.

[7] K. Lundstrom, Viral vectors applied for RNAi-based antiviral therapy, Viruses. (2020). https://doi.org/10.3390/v12090924.

[8] J. Ivan, R. Nurdiansyah, A.A. Parikesit, Computational modeling of AGO-mediated molecular inhibition of ARF6 by miR-145, Indones. J. Biotechnol. 25 (2020). https://doi.org/10.22146/ijbiotech.55631.

[9] P.J. Kaboli, A. Rahmat, P. Ismail, K.-H. Ling, MicroRNA-based therapy and breast cancer: A comprehensive review of novel therapeutic strategies from diagnosis to treatment., Pharmacol. Res. 97 (2015) 104-121. https://doi.org/10.1016/j.phrs.2015.04.015.

[10] M. Fan, R. Krutilina, J. Sun, A. Sethuraman, C.H. Yang, Z.-H. Wu, J. Yue, L.M. Pfeffer, Comprehensive analysis of microRNA (miRNA) targets in breast cancer cells., J. Biol. Chem. 288 (2013) 27480-27493. https://doi.org/10.1074/jbc.M113.491803.

[11] R. Wijaya, A.A. Parikesit, R. Nurdiansyah, 3D And 2D RNA Structure Prediction Of The BRCA2 Gene And Its Silencing RNA In The Breast Cancer, Walisongo J. Chem. 3 (2020) 10. https://doi.org/10.21580/wjc.v3i1.6019.

[12] M. Sahlan, M.N.H. Al Faris, R. Aditama, K. Lischer, A.C. Khayrani, D.K. Pratami, Molecular Docking of South Sulawesi Propolis against Fructose 1,6-Bisphosphatase as a Type 2 Diabetes Mellitus Drug, Int. J. Technol. 11 (2020) 910. https://doi.org/10.14716/ijtech.v11i5.4332.

[13] M. Sahlan, R. Irdiani, D. Flamandita, R. Aditama, S. Alfarraj, M.J. Ansari, A.C. Khayrani, D.K. Pratami, K. Lischer, Molecular interaction analysis of Sulawesi propolis compounds with SARS-CoV-2 main protease as preliminary study for COVID-19 drug discovery., J. King Saud Univ. Sci. 33 (2021) 101234. https://doi.org/10.1016/j.jksus.2020.101234.

[14] A.J. Gandhi, J.D. Rupareliya, V.J. Shukla, S.B. Donga, R. Acharya, An ayurvedic perspective along

with in silico study of the drugs for the management of SARS-CoV-2, J. Ayurveda Integr. Med. (2020). https://doi.org/10.1016/j.jaim.2020.07.002.

[15] M. Amaravani, N.K. Prasad, V. Ramakrishna, COX-2 structural analysis and docking studies with gallic acid structural analogues, Springerplus. (2012). https://doi.org/10.1186/2193-1801-1-58.

[16] R. V. Chikhale, S.K. Sinha, R.B. Patil, S.K. Prasad, A. Shakya, N. Gurav, R. Prasad, S.R. Dhaswadikar, M. Wanjari, S.S. Gurav, In-silico investigation of phytochemicals from Asparagus racemosus as plausible antiviral agent in COVID-19, J. Biomol. Struct. Dyn. (2020). https://doi.org/10.1080/07391102.2020.1784289.

[17] D. Zhang, K. Wu, X. Zhang, S. Deng, B. Peng, In silico screening of Chinese herbal medicines with the potential to directly inhibit 2019 novel coronavirus, J. Integr. Med. 18 (2020) 152-158. https://doi.org/10.1016/j.joim.2020.02.005.

[18] A.A. Parikesit, R. Nurdiansyah, D. Agustriawan, Telaah Sistematis Terhadap Basis Data Bahan Alam untuk Pengembangan Produk Suplemen Herbal, Pros. SEMNASTAN. 0 (2018) 62-68. https://jurnal.umj.ac.id/index.php/semnastan/article/view/2259/1874 (accessed January 28, 2018).

[19] K.E. Hevener, W. Zhao, D.M. Ball, K. Babaoglu, J. Qi, S.W. White, R.E. Lee, Validation of molecular docking programs for virtual screening against dihydropteroate synthase, J. Chem. Inf. Model. 49 (2009) 444-460. https://doi.org/10.1021/ci800293n.

[20] D.T. Moustakas, P.T. Lang, S. Pegg, E. Pettersen, I.D. Kuntz, N. Brooijmans, R.C. Rizzo, Development and validation of a modular, extensible docking program: DOCK 5, J. Comput. Aided. Mol. Des. (2006). https://doi.org/10.1007/s10822-006-9060-4.

[21] A. Setiawati, F.D.O. Riswanto, S.H. Yuliani, E.P. Istyastono, Retrospective Validation of a Structure-Based Virtual Screening Protocol to Identify Ligands for Estrogen Receptor Alpha and Its Application to Identify the Alpha-Mangostin Binding Pose, Indones. J. Chem. 14 (2014) 103-108. https://doi.org/10.22146/ijc.21245.

[22] E.P. Istyastono, F.D.O. Riswanto, S.H. Yuliani, Computer-Aided Drug Repurposing: A Cyclooxygenase-2 Inhibitor Celecoxib as a Ligand for Estrogen Receptor Alpha, Indones. J. Chem. 15 (2015) 274-280. https://doi.org/10.22146/ijc.21196.

[23] A. Radwan, G.M. Mahrous, Docking studies and molecular dynamics simulations of the binding characteristics of waldiomycin and its methyl ester analog to Staphylococcus aureus histidine kinase, PLoS One. 15 (2020) e0234215. https://doi.org/10.1371/journal.pone.0234215.

[24] J. Shamsara, CrossDocker: a tool for performing cross-docking using Autodock Vina, Springerplus. 5 (2016) 344. https://doi.org/10.1186/s40064-016-1972-4.

[25] Z. Ibrahim, B.A. Tejo, M.A.M. Latif, R.A. Karjiban, A.B. Salleh, M.B.A. Rahman, In-silico Identification of Potential Protein Arginine Deiminase IV (PAD4) Inhibitors, Malaysian J. Anal. Sci. 20 (2016) 1269-1277. https://doi.org/10.17576/mjas-2016-2006-05.

[26] M.M. Mysinger, M. Carchia, J.J. Irwin, B.K. Shoichet, Directory of useful decoys, enhanced (DUD-E): Better ligands and decoys for better benchmarking, J. Med. Chem. 55 (2012) 6582-6594. https://doi.org/10.1021/jm300687e.

[27] T. Liu, D. Lu, H. Zhang, M. Zheng, H. Yang, Y. Xu, C. Luo, W. Zhu, K. Yu, H. Jiang, Applying high-performance computing in drug discovery and molecular simulation, Natl. Sci. Rev. 3 (2016) 49-63. https://doi.org/10.1093/nsr/nww003.

[28] H. Zeberg, S. Pääbo, The major genetic risk factor for severe COVID-19 is inherited from Neanderthals, Nature. 587 (2020) 610-612. https://doi.org/10.1038/s41586-020-2818-3.

[29] R. Yuliwulandari, K. Prayuni, R.W. Susilowati, S. Subagyo, S. Soedarsono, A.S. M Sofro, K. Tokunaga, J.G. Shin, NAT2 slow acetylator is associated with anti-tuberculosis drug-induced liver injury severity in Indonesian population, Pharmacogenomics. 20 (2019) 1303-1310. https://doi.org/10.2217/pgs-2019-0131.

[30] M. Fachrul, D.H. Utomo, A.A. Parikesit, lncRNA-based study of epigenetic regulations in diabetic peripheral neuropathy., Silico Pharmacol. 6 (2018) 7. https://doi.org/10.1007/s40203-018-0042-8.

[31] A. Pasipoularides, Genomic translational research: Paving the way to individualized cardiac functional analyses and personalized cardiology, Int. J. Cardiol. 230 (2017) 384-401. https://doi.org/10.1016/j.ijcard.2016.12.097.

[32] S.H. Keenihan, R. Gramzinksi, S. Ratiwayanto, H. Hadiputranto, W. Riberu, S. Soebianto, F. Rusjdy, D. Syafruddin, A. Kartikasari, M. Djojosubroto, I. Setianingsih, A. Harahap, Krisin, D. Fryauff, T. Richie, Y. Charoenvit, H.A. Marwoto, S. Kumar, S. Hoffman, S. Marzuki, K. Baird, *Plasmodium falciparum*: Mechanisms of innate and acquired protection against *Plasmodium falciparum* in Javanese transmigrant adults and children newly resident in malaria-endemic Northwest Papua, in: Adv. Exp. Med. Biol., Kluwer Academic/Plenum Publishers, 2003: pp. 83-102. https://doi.org/10.1007/978-1-4615-0059-9_7.

[33] S. Bernard, D. Agustriawan, Identification of microRNA targeting cancer gene of colorectal carcinoma in Caucasian population, in: 2019 Int. Conf. Inf. Commun. Technol. ICOIACT 2019, Institute of Electrical and Electronics Engineers Inc., 2019: pp. 423-427. https://doi.org/10.1109/ICOIACT46704.2019.8938488.

[34] M.Z. Arifin N, D. Agustriawan, A.A. Parikesit, R. Nurdiansyah, K.N. Ramanto, Identification of microRNAs targeting NAT1 and NAT2 gene transcripts in prostate cancer patients observed in different races, IOP Conf. Ser. Mater. Sci. Eng. 546 (2019) 062017. https://doi.org/10.1088/1757-899X/546/6/062017.

[35] D. Agustriawan, C.H. Huang, J.J.C. Sheu, S.C. Lee, J.J.P. Tsai, N. Kurubanjerdjit, K.L. Ng, DNA methylation-regulated microRNA pathways in ovarian serous cystadenocarcinoma: A meta-analysis, Comput. Biol. Chem. (2016). https://doi.org/10.1016/j.compbiolchem.2016.09.016.

[36] D. Agustriawan, E.B. Wijaya, C.-H. Huang, E. Lim, I.-C. Hsueh, K.-R. Tzeng, K.-L. Ng, MethmiRbase : a Database of DNA Methylation and miRNA Expression in Human Cancer, Lect. Notes Eng. Comput. Sci. I (2016) 16-19.

[37] C.F. Thorn, T.E. Klein, R.B. Altman, Pharmacogenomics and bioinformatics: PharmGKB, Pharmacogenomics. 11 (2010) 501-505. https://doi.org/10.2217/pgs.10.15.

[38] M.D. Luque de Castro, F. Priego-Capote, The analytical process to search for metabolomics biomarkers,

J. Pharm. Biomed. Anal. 147 (2018) 341-349. https://doi.org/10.1016/j.jpba.2017.06.073.

[39] Q. Li, C. Zhao, Y. Zhang, H. Du, T. Xu, X. Xu, J. Zhang, T. Kuang, X. Lai, G. Fan, Y. Zhang, 1H NMR-Based Metabolomics Coupled With Molecular Docking Reveal the Anti-Diabetic Effects and Potential Active Components of Berberis vernae on Type 2 Diabetic Rats, Front. Pharmacol. 11 (2020) 932. https://doi.org/10.3389/fphar.2020.00932.

[40] D.C. Tan, N.K. Kassim, I.S. Ismail, M. Hamid, M.S. Ahamad Bustamam, Identification of antidiabetic metabolites from paederia foetida l. Twigs by gas chromatography-mass spectrometry-based metabolomics and molecular docking study, Biomed Res. Int. 2019 (2019). https://doi.org/10.1155/2019/7603125.

[41] F.C.P. Navarro, H. Mohsen, C. Yan, S. Li, M. Gu, W. Meyerson, M. Gerstein, Genomics and data science: An application within an umbrella, Genome Biol. 20 (2019) 109. https://doi.org/10.1186/s13059-019-1724-1.

[42] J. Godzien, A. Gil de la Fuente, A. Otero, C. Barbas, Metabolite Annotation and Identification, in: Compr. Anal. Chem., Elsevier B.V., 2018: pp. 415-445. https://doi.org/10.1016/bs.coac.2018.07.004.

[43] L. Ang, E. Song, H.W. Lee, M.S. Lee, Herbal Medicine for the Treatment of Coronavirus Disease 2019 (COVID-19): A Systematic Review and Meta-Analysis of Randomized Controlled Trials, J. Clin. Med. 9 (2020) 1583. https://doi.org/10.3390/jcm9051583.

[44] X. Luo, X. Ni, J. Lin, Y. Zhang, L. Wu, D. Huang, Y. Liu, J. Guo, W. Wen, Y. Cai, Y. Chen, L. Lin, The add-on effect of Chinese herbal medicine on COVID-19: A systematic review and meta-analysis, Phytomedicine. (2020) 153282. https://doi.org/10.1016/j.phymed.2020.153282.

[45] W. Pang, Z. Liu, N. Li, Y. Li, F. Yang, B. Pang, X. Jin, W. Zheng, J. Zhang, Chinese medical drugs for coronavirus disease 2019: a systematic review and meta-analysis, Integr. Med. Res. 9 (2020) 100477. https://doi.org/10.1016/j.imr.2020.100477.

[46] S. Vaishya, R.D. Sarwade, V. Seshadri, MicroRNA, proteins, and metabolites as novel biomarkers for prediabetes, diabetes, and related complications, Front. Endocrinol. (Lausanne). 9 (2018). https://doi.org/10.3389/fendo.2018.00180.

[47] F. Anwar, H.N. Altayb, F.A. Al-Abbasi, A.L. Al-Malki, M.A. Kamal, V. Kumar, Antiviral effects of probiotic metabolites on COVID-19., J. Biomol. Struct. Dyn. (2020) 1-10. https://doi.org/10.1080/07391102.2020.1775123.

[48] H. Refaat, F.M. Mady, H.A. Sarhan, H.S. Rateb, E. Alaaeldin, Optimization and evaluation of propolis liposomes as a promising therapeutic approach for COVID-19, Int. J. Pharm. (2020). https://doi.org/10.1016/j.ijpharm.2020.120028.

[49] C.A. Scorza, V.C. Gonçalves, F.A. Scorza, A.C. Fiorini, A.C.G. de Almeida, M.C.M. Fonseca, J. Finsterer, Propolis and coronavirus disease 2019 (COVID-19): Lessons from nature, Complement. Ther. Clin. Pract. 41 (2020) 101227. https://doi.org/10.1016/j.ctcp.2020.101227.

[50] A.A. Berretta, M.A.D. Silveira, J.M. Cóndor Capcha, D. De Jong, Propolis and its potential against SARS-CoV-2 infection mechanisms and COVID-19 disease: Running title: Propolis against SARS-CoV-2 infection and COVID-19, Biomed. Pharmacother. 131 (2020) 110622. https://doi.org/10.1016/j.biopha.2020.110622.

[51] H.I. Güler, G. Tatar, O. Yildiz, A.O. Belduz, ..., An investigation of ethanolic propolis extracts: Their potential inhibitor properties against ACE-II receptors for COVID-19 treatment by Molecular Docking Study, Sci. .... (2020).

[52] A. Amit Koparde, R. Chandrashekar Doijad, C. Shripal Magdum, Natural Products in Drug Discovery, in: Pharmacogn. - Med. Plants, IntechOpen, 2019. https://doi.org/10.5772/intechopen.82860.

[53] A. Fadholly, A.N.M. Ansori, T.H. Sucipto, An overview of naringin: Potential anticancer compound of citrus fruits, Res. J. Pharm. Technol. 13 (2020) 5613-5619. https://doi.org/10.5958/0974-360X.2020.00979.8.

[54] W.E. Putra, V.D. Kharisma, H. Susanto, Potential of *Zingiber officinale* bioactive compounds as inhibitory agent against the IKK-B, in: AIP Conf. Proc., American Institute of Physics Inc., 2020: p. 040048. https://doi.org/10.1063/5.0002478.

[55] V. Dhea Kharisma, A. Nur, M. Ansori, A. Fadholly, T.H. Sucipto, Molecular Mechanism of Caffeine-Aspirin Interaction in Kopi Balur 1 as Anti-Inflammatory Agent: A Computational Study, 2020. https://doi.org/10.37506/IJFMT.V14I4.12274.

[56] World Health Organization, Global Report on Diabetes, Isbn. 978 (2016) 88. https://doi.org/ISBN 978 92 4 156525 7.

[57] C. Guay, R. Regazzi, Circulating microRNAs as novel biomarkers for diabetes mellitus, Nat. Rev. Endocrinol. 9 (2013) 513-521. https://doi.org/10.1038/nrendo.2013.86.

[58] E. Guarino, C.D. Poggi, G.E. Grieco, V. Cenci, E. Ceccarelli, I. Crisci, G. Sebastiani, F. Dotta, Circulating MicroRNAs as biomarkers of gestational diabetes mellitus: Updates and perspectives, Int. J. Endocrinol. 2018 (2018). https://doi.org/10.1155/2018/6380463.

[59] M. Frédérich, B. Pirotte, M. Fillet, P. De Tullio, Metabolomics as a Challenging Approach for Medicinal Chemistry and Personalized Medicine, J. Med. Chem. 59 (2016) 8649-8666. https://doi.org/10.1021/acs.jmedchem.5b01335.

[60] L. Li, R. Li, J. Zhou, A. Zuniga, A.E. Stanislaus, Y. Wu, T. Huan, J. Zheng, Y. Shi, D.S. Wishart, G. Lin, MyCompoundID: Using an evidence-based metabolome library for metabolite identification, Anal. Chem. 85 (2013) 3401-3408. https://doi.org/10.1021/ac400099b.

[61] A. Yanuar, A. Mun'im, A.B.A. Lagho, R.R. Syahdi, M. Rahmat, H. Suhartanto, Medicinal Plants Database and Three Dimensional Structure of the Chemical Compounds from Medicinal Plants in Indonesia, Int. J. Comput. Sci. 8 (2011) 180-183. http://arxiv.org/abs/1111.7183 (accessed March 23, 2014).

[62] A.A. Parikesit, B. Ardiansah, D.M. Handayani, U.S.F. Tambunan, D. Kerami, Virtual screening of Indonesian flavonoid as neuraminidase inhibitor of influenza a subtype H5N1, IOP Conf. Ser. Mater. Sci. Eng. 107 (2016) 012053. https://doi.org/10.1088/1757-899X/107/1/012053.

[63] D.S. Wishart, C. Knox, A.C. Guo, S. Shrivastava, M. Hassanali, P. Stothard, Z. Chang, J. Woolsey, DrugBank: a comprehensive resource for in silico drug discovery and exploration., Nucleic Acids Res. 34 (2006) D668–D672.

[64] S. Kim, P.A. Thiessen, E.E. Bolton, J. Chen, G. Fu, A. Gindulyte, L. Han, J. He, S. He, B.A. Shoemaker, J. Wang, B. Yu, J. Zhang, S.H. Bryant, PubChem substance and compound databases,

Nucleic Acids Res. 44 (2016) D1202–D1213. https://doi.org/10.1093/nar/gkv951.

[65] M. Kanehisa, M. Furumichi, M. Tanabe, Y. Sato, K. Morishima, KEGG: New perspectives on genomes, pathways, diseases and drugs, Nucleic Acids Res. 45 (2017) D353–D361. https://doi.org/10.1093/nar/gkw1092.

[66] T. Wang, M.-B. Wu, Z.-J. Chen, H. Chen, J.-P. Lin, L.-R. Yang, Fragment-based drug discovery and molecular docking in drug design., Curr. Pharm. Biotechnol. 16 (2015) 11-25. http://www.ncbi.nlm.nih.gov/pubmed/25420726 (accessed February 24, 2015).

[67] Y. Chen, D.T. Pohlhaus, In silico docking and scoring of fragments., Drug Discov. Today. Technol. 7 (2010) e147–e202. https://doi.org/10.1016/j.ddtec.2010.11.002.

[68] D. Seebach, Organic Synthesis—Where now?, Angew. Chemie Int. Ed. English. 29 (1990) 1320-1367. https://doi.org/10.1002/anie.199013201.

[69] R. Liu, X. Li, K.S. Lam, Combinatorial chemistry in drug discovery, Curr. Opin. Chem. Biol. 38 (2017) 117-126. https://doi.org/10.1016/j.cbpa.2017.03.017.

[70] H. Zhang, Y. Xu, P. Jia, Y. Zhu, G. Zhang, J. Zhang, S. Duan, W. Kang, T. Wang, R. Jing, J. Cheng, Y. Liu, Q. Yang, Global trends of antimicrobial susceptibility to ceftaroline and ceftazidime–avibactam: a surveillance study from the ATLAS program (2012-2016), Antimicrob. Resist. Infect. Control. 9 (2020) 166. https://doi.org/10.1186/s13756-020-00829-z.

[71] C.L. Gargalo, I. Udugama, K. Pontius, P.C. Lopez, R.F. Nielsen, A. Hasanzadeh, S.S. Mansouri, C. Bayer, H. Junicke, K. V. Gernaey, Towards smart biomanufacturing: a perspective on recent developments in industrial measurement and monitoring technologies for bio-based production processes, J. Ind. Microbiol. Biotechnol. 47 (2020) 947-964. https://doi.org/10.1007/s10295-020-02308-1.

[72] A. Boulila, M. Ayadi, S. Marzouki, S. Bouzidi, Contribution to a biomedical component production using incremental sheet forming, Int. J. Adv. Manuf. Technol. 95 (2018) 2821-2833. https://doi.org/10.1007/s00170-017-1397-4.

[73] M.F.A.-H. Ginoga, R. Trisminingsih, W.A. Kusuma, Drug-Target Visualization on IJAH Analytics Using Sankey Diagram, in: 2020 Int. Conf. Comput. Sci. Its Appl. Agric., IEEE, 2020: pp. 1-6. https://doi.org/10.1109/ICOSICA49951.2020.9243285.

[74] A. Reinaldo, W.A. Kusuma, H. Rahmawan, Y. Herdiyeni, Implementation of Breadth-First Search Parallel to Predict Drug-Target Interaction in Plant-Disease Graph, in: 2020 Int. Conf. Comput. Sci. Its Appl. Agric., IEEE, 2020: pp. 1-5. https://doi.org/10.1109/ICOSICA49951.2020.9243216.

[75] D. Afdhal, K.W. Ananta, W.S. Hartono, Adverse Drug Reactions Prediction Using Multi-label Linear Discriminant Analysis and Multi-label Learning, 2020 Int. Conf. Adv. Comput. Sci. Inf. Syst. (2020) 69-76. https://doi.org/10.1109/ICACSIS51025.2020.9263166.

[76] F. Sulistiawan, W.A. Kusuma, N.S. Ramadhanti, A. Tedjo, Drug-Target Interaction Prediction in Coronavirus Disease 2019 Case Using Deep Semi-Supervised Learning Model, in: 2020 Int. Conf. Adv. Comput. Sci. Inf. Syst., IEEE, 2020: pp. 83-88. https://doi.org/10.1109/ICACSIS51025.2020.9263241.

[77] S. Dash, S.K. Shakyawar, M. Sharma, S. Kaushik, Big data in healthcare: management, analysis and future prospects, J. Big Data. 6 (2019) 1-25. https://doi.org/10.1186/s40537-019-0217-0.

[78] D. Besozzi, L. Manzoni, M.S. Nobile, S. Spolaor, M. Castelli, L. Vanneschi, P. Cazzaniga, S. Ruberto, L. Rundo, A. Tangherloni, Computational Intelligence for Life Sciences, Fundam. Informaticae. 171 (2019) 57-80. https://doi.org/10.3233/FI-2020-1872.

[79] A.A. PARIKESIT, D. ANUROGO, R.A. PUTRANTO, Pemanfaatan bioinformatika dalam bidang pertanian dan kesehatan (The utilization of bioinformatics in the field of agriculture and health), E-Journal Menara Perkeb. 85 (2017). https://doi.org/10.22302/iribb.jur.mp.v85i2.237.

[80] F.H. Hasanah, E. Sulistyaningsih, W.D. Sawitri, The Expression of The PfEMP1-DBL2β Recombinant Protein of Plasmodium falciparum Welch, 1897 Isolated From Indonesia, J. ILMU DASAR. 21 (2020) 67. https://doi.org/10.19184/jid.v21i1.10494.

[81] A.A. Parikesit, D.H. Utomo, N. Karimah, Protein Domain Annotation of Plasmodium spp. Circumsporozoite Protein (CSP) Using Hidden Markov Model-based Tools, J. Biol. Indones. 14 (2018) 185-190. https://doi.org/10.14203/jbi.v14i2.3737.

[82] N. Tomar, R.K. De, Immunoinformatics: an integrated scenario, Immunology. 131 (2010) 153-168. https://doi.org/10.1111/j.1365-2567.2010.03330.x.

[83] D.R. Flower, Immunoinformatics: Predicting Immunogenicity in Silico, Humana, 2007. http://books.google.co.id/books?id=IJtZurJ5BvoC.

Chapter 2

Pharmacogenomics: Overview, Applications, and Recent Developments

Rahul Shukla

Abstract

Pharmacogenomics is defined as the study of genes and how an individual response is affected due to drugs. Pharmacogenomics is an emerging new branch with combination of both pharmacology (the branch of science that deals with study of drugs) as well as genomics (the branch of science that deals with study of genes) for development of effective doses and safe medications tailored according an individual patient genetic makeup. Human Genome Project is one of the crucial projects in which researchers are developing and learning relation in genes and its effect on the body's response to medications. Difference in genetic makeup provides difference in effectiveness of medication and in future to predict effectiveness of medication for an individual and to study existence of adverse drug reactions. Besides advancement in the field of science and technology till date pharmacogenomics hangs in infancy. There is limited use of pharmacogenomics, but still, novel approaches are under clinical trials. In near future, pharmacogenomics will enable development of tailor-made therapeutics for treating widespread health problems like neurodegenerative, cardiovascular disorders, HIV, cancer, asthma, etc.

Keywords: pharmacogenomics, genomics, proteomics, personalized medicines, tailored drugs

1. Pharmacogenomics: overview

Due to variability existence among individuals against drug therapy response, it is a challenging task to predict the degree of effectiveness of a medication to a particular patient. As we know various clinical factors which are known to affect drug response, for example body size, age, sex, hepatic and renal function, and associated drug use (**Table 1**). Along with these clinical factors, some pharmacological factors also play a major role which includes differences in metabolism, drug distribution and drug directed proteins [2, 3]. Recently, major causes of interindividual differences are shown by variations in genes encoding cytochrome P450 (CYP) and other metabolizing enzymes in plasma concentrations of some drugs [4, 5].

Pharmacogenetics and pharmacogenomics can be used interchangeably. Though, Pharmacogenomics refers to the whole range of genes that are related to the determination of drug efficacy and safety whereas pharmacogenetics means monogenetic variants which alter the drug response [6, 7]. Pharmacogenomics is defined as study of genes and how they affect an individual response to the

Factors	Effects
a. **Genetic factors**	
Drug-metabolizing enzymes	Drug metabolism (pharmacokinetics)
Therapeutic targets	Drug efficacy (pharmacodynamics)
Targets of ADRs	Drug toxicity
Drug transporters	Drug disposition
b. **Environmental factors**	
Environmental chemicals, alcohol drinking, combined drugs effect, and dietary substances	Drug efficacy, toxicity, and pharmacokinetics
c. **Physiological factors**	
Age, sex, pregnancy, exercise, disease state, starvation	Drug efficacy, toxicity, and pharmacokinetics

Table 1.
Genome-wide association studies in pharmacogenomics [1].

administered drugs. Pharmacogenomics is emerging new branch with combination of both pharmacology (branch of science which deals with study of drugs) as well as genomics (the branch of science which deals with study of genes) for development of effective doses and safe medications tailored according an individual patient genetic makeup (**Figure 1**) [8, 9].

Basically, the concept for pharmacogenetics was left unknown for more than 50 years. This study underlined to the molecular mechanisms in account for their variation in responses to drug due to inherited characters and in drug development process. Pharmacogenomics applications can be employed in the improvement of discovery of new entities and its development with two possible ways: target the new drug targets or development of new entity to overcome drug resistance, and another way is to optimize the pharmacokinetics and metabolism of drug for reduction of the drug level variations [10]. In fact, personalized drug therapy or individualized drug therapy is not an easy task. It needs many folds as there may be a lack of information regarding drug action, genomic elements of important disease pathogenesis, especially for complex diseases. Also, large scale clinical studies are sometimes becoming a big challenge for the researchers [11]. The correlation of pharmacogenomics and cancer would expand the specific anticancer drugs with better chemotherapeutic outcomes [12–15]. There are prominent examples with recent clinical and pharmaceutical restrains where the molecular based mechanisms are involved in various drug responses were observed among the patients and diagnosed with the similar diseases [16, 17]. Moreover, various polymorphisms existence at genetic levels in genes found to have association with alteration in responses of drug and rate of ADRs in humans (**Table 2**) [18].

Finally, pharmacogenomics-based development of drug and its regulation will open the doors for new as well as targeted drug development for promoting safe, effective, and cost-effective drug therapy for individual. The theoretical origin for pharmacogenomics is outlined by Sir Archibald Garrod's in book entitled as "1939 Inborn Factors of Disease" [19].

Pharmacogenetics is the study of how an individual person's genes respond to a drug. This branch is associated with genomics is genetic level studies with functional studies and pharmacology (includes pharmacokinetics and pharmacodynamics). All these branches together aid in the development of safe, and effective medications along with doses which are probably tailored to an individual persona genetic makeup [20–24]. Pharmacogenetics is indicated as major clinically proven

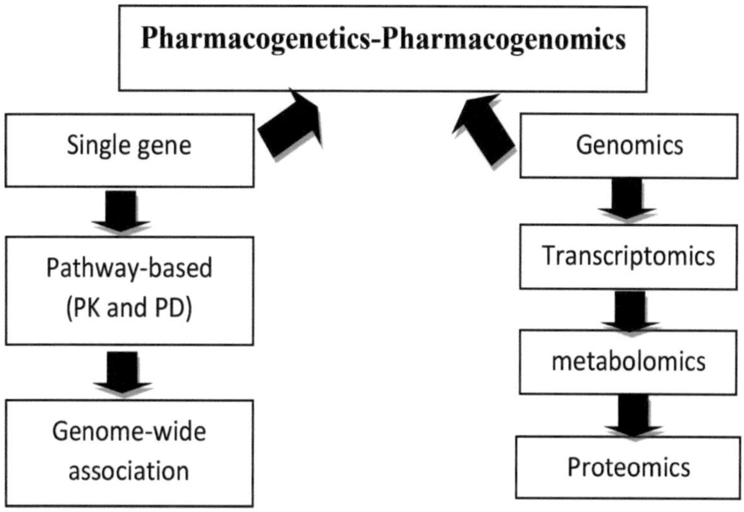

Figure 1.
Development of pharmacogenomics and pharmacogenetics.

Polymorphic gene	Drug	Effect
CYP2C9	Phenytoin	Toxicity
	Warfarin	Bleeding risk
	Glipizide	Hypoglycaemia
TPMT	Anticancer drugs like 6-thiopurine, 6-Mercaptopurine, azathioprine	Toxicity
Human leukocyte antigens (HLA)	Abacavir	Related to hypersensitivity
N-acetyltransferase (NATs)	Sulphonamides, hydralazine, Isoniazid	Toxicity, hypersensitivity
UDP-glucuronosyltransferase 1A1 (UGT1A1)	Irinotecan	Toxicity
CYP2D6	Codeine	Toxicity
	Fluoxetine	Toxicity
MDRI	Antiepileptic drugs	Drug response

Table 2.
Genes with altered drug response.

application in terms of advancement in human genomic science. This potentiates a revolution in drug therapy. As a result, diseases which range from depression to viral infection and from childhood leukemia to hypertension are treated or controlled for enhancing the quality of life of patient. Most medicines at present are available as "one medication fits all" but they sometimes were not capable to work same to everyone. So, it is difficult to envisage who will have benefit result and who will have negative side effects. Also, the knowledge which scientist have acquired due to extensive work on Human Genome Project and are learning about inherited variations of genes and there effect on body's response to medications. Conditions in which responses of an individual to certain drugs include Stevens-Johnson syndrome or epidermal toxic necrolysis, clopidogrel resistance, malignant hyperthermia, warfarin sensitivity and its resistance and thiopurine S-methyltransferase deficiency [25].

2. Application

Many common diseases having high morbidity as well as mortality rates have now known with well-established genetic components. The degree of role of genetics has been predicted for diseases like obesity and diabetes according to their sibling analysis [26, 27]. In the same way, some rare gene mutations can provide a vision into the more complex biological processes [28]. For instance, when the subject possesses extreme levels of HDL in their blood, one can easily demonstrated the influence of CETP (cholesteryl ester transfer protein) on patients HDL levels [29–31]. In another case, a person having deactivating mutations due to the Janus kinase 3 (JAK 3) gene shows severe combination of immune-deficient syndrome, as sometimes inhibition of JAK3 was expected to affect the human immune suppression [32, 33]. Hence, this led to a new investigation on drugs having CETP inhibition and JAK3 inhibition with the help of pharmacogenetics [34]. Also, with the advent of pharmacogenomics, the path of relationships between disease state and human genes has now established which led to the suitable selection of therapeutic targets.

Nowadays, many academic institutions and Pharmaceutical companies are moving toward the investigation on the relationship between disease phenotypes and genetic variations to better categorize diseases [35, 36]. Although the collection of medical phenotypes having linkages with samples of DNA provides a prominent opportunity for examine the genetic variation which are present in patients. Investigation of genetic variation can be done by collection of DNA of particular patient. This is characterized in a study where DNA from a person involves in trails of lipid lowering demonstrated a swift connection between phenotypic novel lipase gene family and for HDL levels. As per literature reports, above mentioned studies are based on a sound hypothesis which is linked to candidate's biological gene selection. Now it is easy to cross-examine the genome selection which is solely depends on phenotypic criteria [10, 37]. These stages have now substituted around 300,000 SNPs across the genome, by exploiting only few haplotype-defining SNPs. Perlegen sciences have developed newly genotyping technologies which has with a capability of genotyping mass hundreds or thousands of markers with the help of high-density based oligonucleotide arrays linked with restriction enzyme-based genomic reduction. However, as these technologies advances, still exact number of haplotype-defining SNPs is uncertain. Some findings are recently reported relation to assess polymorphisms across selected gene regions recommends that, it is necessary to reach an r^2 of >0.8% in order to detect more than 80% of all haplotypes. Due to HapMap project progression with defined LD patterns linkage, scientist working on genes will thorough assess to the degree of LD in a represented regions or selected regions. This will enable to explore more around selection of SNP regardless design of study [38, 39]. As genome approach does not depend upon selection of candidate genes, so understanding on complex diseases such as psychiatric or cardiovascular diseases will become more efficient. Some researchers believed that the new horizons on LD coverage about insights of human genome and SNP density will show the perception of a substantial genomic portion areas and its relation with interest of phenotype [40, 41]. To assess the Perlegen Sciences chip-based array-based platform and to justify the haplotype tagging approach for the identification of genetic associations, 7283 SNPs connecting 17.1 mega bases (Mb) of DNA were genotyped for detecting linkages with HDL levels. Further, SNPs were connected with 50 CETP haploblock gene were found out as the most valuable association in dataset. The companies like Perlegen and project like Hap Map project recently declared their purpose to provide it SNPs markers into public provinces to further advent to basis for such kind of experiments which help in the scientific community [42, 43].

Pharmacogenetics significantly expands the therapy outcomes and drug uses. Medications may prescribe in low dose under strict monitoring to patients which shows genetically predisposed to their adverse events. This would probably helpful for drugs having narrow therapeutic index such as warfarin may be started gradually in patients having VKORC1 genotype linked with improved warfarin sensitivity. With the help of pharmacogenetics, it is now possible to reduce the number of subjects to conduct any experiment and chances of error may be eliminated for many diseases [44, 45].

On the contrary, clinicians may be able to minimize possible adverse effects with the aid of genetic information for matching suitable drug to suitable patient at an appropriate dose. For instances, traditional approach to the management of hypertension involves the trial of numerous anti-hypertensive drugs till the desired blood pressure achieved with adequate drug tolerability. In this case, few initial drugs/agents fail to produce lower blood pressure or shown intolerable adverse effects. This way of selection of drugs took long time which ultimately suffered by patients. On the contrary, Pharmacogenetics, based on the patients' DNA, offers the greatest response with the best tolerability of the drug. Based on genetic regulator of cellular functions, pharmacogenetics may be able to produce new drugs with less adverse effects. For example, chromosome translocation and its derived enzymes are responsible for causing life-threatening chronic myeloid leukemia (CML) which led to accelerate FDA approval of inhibitor of translocation-created enzyme Imatinib [46]. In the end, this core subject improves the quality and cut-down the total costs of healthcare by minimizing the number of adverse reaction and reduce treatment failures gives rise to the discovery of new genetic targets for disease management [47–49].

3. Case studies

3.1 Thiopurine therapy and TPMT (thiopurine methyltransferase) testing

Thiopurine are the categories of drugs that are used to conquer the normal activity of the body's immune system. In short, these are called antimetabolites chiefly used as an antiproliferative as well as immunosuppressants such as mercaptopurine and azathioprine. 6-mercaptopurine daily administered for 3–4 years for treating childhood leukemia, while azathioprine which is a prodrug of 6-mercaptopurine prescribed for treating inflammatory bowel disease (also known as Crohn's disease) [50]. TPMT methylates thiopurine compounds. S-adenosyl-L-methionine acts as methyl donor and converts it into S-adenosyl-L-homocysteine [51, 52]. So, TPMT metabolizes various thiopurine based drugs with mechanism of S-adenosyl-L-methionine while S-methyl acting as donor, while S-adenosyl-L-homocysteine acting as a derivative. Genetic polymorphism which affects basically enzymatic activity has association with variations in toxicity and sensitivity within individuals due to such drugs. Nearby 1/300 individual is lacking for this enzyme. TPMT has not recognized to have any phenotype in the absence of encounter drug. TPMT is now enlists by FDA as a pharmacogenomic biomarker for various adverse drug reactions related to cisplatin such as cisplatin-induced ototoxicity in teenagers [47, 53–55].

Patients having identical alleles at equivalent chromosomal loci accumulate unnecessary thioguanine nucleotides levels (up to 10-fold higher related with wild types) and treatment with standard dosages of drug and leading to a hematopoietic toxicity (pancytopenia and myelosuppression) which is life-threatening condition [56, 57].

In more concise way, patients having heterozygous gene variations are also at high risk in terms of toxicity and dosage reductions is prior in these cases up to their tolerate therapy. According to pharmacoeconomic studies, the determination of the TPMT genotype is cost-effective and it must be checked prior to the start of therapy. According to a review of the literature, it was found that TPMT testing with clinical performances for myelosuppression was estimated with specificity of 89%, sensitivity of 32%, 9% PPV and NPV of 97% (**Table 3**). The low estimated value represents low incidence of severity in myelosuppression especially in those patients who are carrier of not less than one defective allele. Researchers have estimated the net cost for avoidance of serious events of myelosuppression. Out of 1000 patients receiving azathioprine, only 3.2% (equivalent to 32 cases) have founded with severe leukopenia and TPMT screening avoided as third of those trials [50, 58].

Iorio and co-workers have analyzed drug responses on various human cancer cell lines. The mapping was done for around 11K tumors obtained from different 29 different human tissues as per Cancer of Genome Atlas (TCGA) enlisted from 1000 cancer cell lines as per Genomics of Drug Sensitivity in Cancer resource. In another event, TCGA patient gene expression was studied for drug response. In this, more than 140 gene drug interactions were studied with specific somatic biomarkers [59–61].

3.2 Abacavir therapy and HLA testing

Abacavir which is HIV-1 nucleoside with reverse transcriptase inhibition is employed for management of HIV/AIDS. It is well tolerated but sometimes shows common to more severe side-effects which include lactic acidosis, hypersensitivity [62]. In some studies, it was observed that a genetic testing/marker can help in predicting whether a HIV-infected patient is at high risk of abacavir induced severe hypersensitivity reactions (approx. 5% of patients) [63, 64]. This hypersensitivity reaction accompanies with lethal gastrointestinal symptoms, rashes, and fever. This reaction is life threatening, particularly if drug is restarted and discontinued. One study has shown about an occurrence of human leukocyte antigen (HLA) B05701 is main cause of hypersensitivity [45, 65]. Based on the Australian cohort, patients were 114 times more hypersensitivity due to HLA-B5701 allele reaction, whereas in an industry-sponsored study revealed that patients with the HLA-B5701 allele was associated with 24 times more likely to experience of hypersensitivity reaction [45]. Thus, one way to solve this issue is genetic testing which integrates pharmacogenetics into the clinical practice. The distribution of HLA-B5701 allele can be detected in many worldwide populations (**Table 4**).

3.3 Statin therapy and polymorphic angiotensin-converting enzyme

Statins (HMGCoA) reductase inhibitors most often used in management of hypercholesterolemia condition accompanying with elevation in risk to coronary heart disease [66, 67]. Due to increased number of cases of hypercholesterolemia along with volume of statins related prescriptions in US, it creates a significant interest in optimization of costs related to these therapies [31]. Recent investigations have told that polymorphism in I/D angiotensin converting enzyme (ACE) has correlation with risk of heart related syndromes in men when treated with statins [68–70]. Next 2 years of statin medication, in which males who are having DD genotype (equivalent to 27% of patients) shown to have no effect on the risk of coronary heart disease (with relative risk factor of 1.34), in comparison to males with ID (equivalent to 21% of patients) present a marked decreased in risk of coronary cardiovascular disease (with relative risk rate of 0.87), II genotype

Clinical performances	(%)
Percent responders	40.0
Sensitivity	75.0
Specificity	66.7
Frequency mutation	50.0
Positive predictive value (PPV)	60.0
Negative predictive value (PPV)	80.0

Table 3.
Clinical performances of the test.

Population group	HLA-B5701 carrier frequency range (%)
Asian	00–6.5
Southwest Asian	4–19.5
Middle Eastern	0.5–6.2
African	0.0–3.5
European	1.5–10.5
Mexican	0.0–4.2
South American	1.2–3.2

Table 4.
Allele frequency of HLA-B5701 allele in various population groups.

(equivalent to 22% of patients) having relative risk of 0.23, thus concluding that patients bearing DD genotype did not take advantages from statin treatment. Also, testing of I/D genotype might results in cost effective as few patients presents the I/I or I/D genotype [70].

3.4 Muscle relaxant succinylcholine and antitubercular drug, INH

These two conventional illustrations of pharmacogenetics involve the genetic variation along with enzymatic metabolism (enzymatic hydrolysis and acetylation). Both act as a monogenic trait and involved PK variations because of inheritance differences [71, 72]. It was observed that some patients with succinylcholine treatment experienced a serious and lethal adverse event i.e. prolonged muscle paralysis which is due to inherited "atypical" butyryl cholinesterase enzyme (BCHE). Later, it was established that BCHE allele which encodes the most usual atypical form of enzyme comprised with a nonsynonymous coding i.e. single nucleotide polymorphism (nSNP), G209 > A, results in Asp70 > Gly change in encoded amino acid which altered active sites of enzyme [73, 74]. But atypical BCHE has less ability to catalyze the succinylcholine hydrolysis and could resist to inhibition due to dibucaine compound [37, 75].

Tuberculosis is the most problematic disease of both developing as well as under-developed nations. The conformity to patients with tuberculosis is due to common lethal adverse reactions and supposed to have important aspect providing high prevalence [76, 77]. Many investigations showed that the polymorphisms of N-acetyl transferase 2 (NAT-2), CYP2E1 as well as glutathione S transferase (GST-1) would be able to influence concentration of liver toxic isoniazid metabolites in plasma. Some polymorphic genes contribute in the INH induced hepatotoxicity by altering the anti-oxidant enzyme expression, these gene polymorphisms include glucuronosyltransferase (UGT), basic region of leucine zipper factor family (CNC) homolo (BACH), human leukocyte antigen (HLA), nitric oxide synthase (NOS) and Maf basic leucine zipper protein (MAFK). Till date the above mentioned studies encounter with many limitations [77–79].

3.5 Warfarin

Warfarin is a medication that is commonly used as an anticoagulant which means blood thinner. It aids in treating blood clots such as pulmonary embolism and deep vein thrombosis, and to prevent heart diseases associated with clotting. It has very narrow therapeutic index [80, 81]. However, warfarin therapy may result in complicated adverse reactions including both coagulation and hemorrhage. The racemic mixture of warfarin, S-form is 3–5 times more potent in comparison to R-form of an anticoagulant, and easily gets metabolized due to genetically polymorphic CYP450 isoform i.e. CYP2C9 [82]. CYP2C9 exists in two common polymorphic form, Arg144 > Cys (CYP2C9*2) as well as Ile358 > Leu (CYP2C9*3) modifications in coded sequence of amino acid, with nearly 12 and 5%, respectively. These forms vary between 8 and 10% in Caucasians, with minor occurrence in subject from Southeast Asia. A report in 1999, which confirms patients with one or two common CYP2C9 variant alleles, requires a "low" warfarin dose. These subjects had a risen risk of hemorrhage during warfarin therapy. In 2004, the gene encoded targeting VKORC1 (vitamin K epoxide reductase complex 1) was cloned. In a study, it was found that patients with VKORC1 type of haplotypes requires low dose, the average warfarin maintenance dose was nearly half for subjects with haplotypes having high dose maintenance. In this study, the grouping of both VKORC1 haplotyping as well as genotyping for CYP2C9 described around 25% of dose variance in warfarin. Other studies reported similar results in 2005. The Pharmacogenetics Knowledge Base (PharmGKB), in which data base is reinforced by the National Institutes of Health (NIH) along with part of the NIH Pharmacogenetics Research Network (PGRN), originated an association for consolidation of warfarin pharmacogenetic data throughout the world [83, 84]. In this evaluation of variation in genetic drug target as well as drug metabolism if and only if when VKORC1 and CYP2C9 haplotypes were determined. The figure demonstrates a schematic illustration of both pharmacokinetic (CYP2C9-dependent) as well as pharmacodynamic (VKORC1-dependent) pharmacogenomic aspects that effects final dose of warfarin (**Figure 2**).

It is important to know that by identifying the individual genetic properties, we can improve the dosing of warfarin. In general, VKORC1 haplotypes have three-fold greater effect on an individual's warfarin dose than CYP2C9. Both can play a vital role in the potential for estimating the therapeutic warfarin dose. In August 2007, FDA approved a change in labeling of warfarin package stating, "lower starting doses should be considered for patients with some genetic alterations in VKORC1 and CYP2C9 enzymes" [80].

4. Outlook

These cases prove that patient care could be improved effectively by pharmacogenetic based approaches. Although, the allelic occurrences of the gene alterations must be visibly defined in the subjects studied must be well established. Out of above-mentioned cases, no one is absolute, so it is better to perform the sensitivity analyses as well as to regulate the robustness of conclusion with variation in probabilities [85, 86]. Move onward, it is utmost important for maintaining the possible

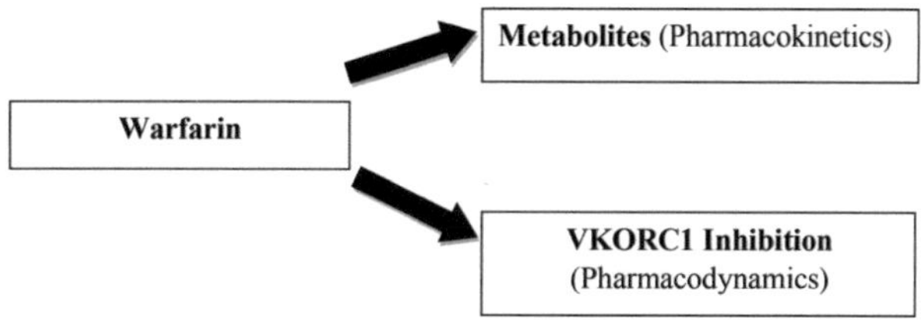

Figure 2.
Warfarin pharmacogenomics.

cost-effectiveness of few recently published pharmacogenetic associated reports, for instance, vitamin K epoxide reductase gene variants envisage the warfarin response [87–89]. Lastly, it will be significant to collect pharmacoeconomic and pharmacogenetic statistics together during industry-funded clinical trials for bringing cost effective theragnostic in a sensible manner [90, 91].

5. Conclusion

Individualized therapeutics or tailor-made therapy is one of the major goals of pharmacogenomics. In relation to inheritance other factors also contribute to individual therapeutics due to variation in response to administration of drug. Recently many developments in the field of pharmacology and genomics have made possible for physicians to achieve individualization of therapeutics. These recent developments create possibility of thorough basis of particular drug for particular patient with motive of tailor-made therapy. Futuristic development in field of pharmacogenomics has paved the way to new emerging fields of pharmacoproteomic, pharmacotranscriptomics, and pharmacometabolomic. These new branches of science make it possible to achieve the concept of treat each patient as unique, complex, fascinating individual. At the end doubts about achieving individualized therapeutics with the help of this integrated system is still a dream in 21st century era.

Acknowledgements

The NIPER-R communication number for this manuscript is NIPER-R/Communication/156.

Conflict of interest

The authors declare no conflict of interest among themselves.

Author details

Rahul Shukla
Department of Pharmaceutics, National Institute of Pharmaceutical Education and Research (NIPER)-Raebareli, Lucknow, Uttar Pradesh, India

*Address all correspondence to: rahulshuklapharm@gmail.com

References

[1] Daly AK. Genome-wide association studies in pharmacogenomics. Nature Reviews. Genetics. 2010;**11**(4):241-246

[2] Caldwell MD, Berg RL, Zhang KQ, Glurich I, Schmelzer JR, Yale SH, et al. Evaluation of genetic factors for warfarin dose prediction. Clinical Medicine & Research. 2007;**5**(1):8-16

[3] Wattanachai N, Kaewmoongkun S, Pussadhamma B, Makarawate P, Wongvipaporn C, Kiatchoosakun S, et al. The impact of non-genetic and genetic factors on a stable warfarin dose in Thai patients. European Journal of Clinical Pharmacology. 2017;**73**(8):973-980

[4] Cha PC, Zembutsu H, Takahashi A, Kubo M, Kamatani N, Nakamura Y. A genome-wide association study identifies SNP in DCC is associated with gallbladder cancer in the Japanese population. Journal of Human Genetics. 2012;**57**(4):235-237

[5] Chadwick R, Ten Have H, Meslin EM. The Sage Handbook of Health Care Ethics. Sage Publications; 2011

[6] Alsanosi SM, Skiffington C, Padmanabhan S. Pharmacokinetic pharmacogenomics. In: Handbook of Pharmacogenomics and Stratified Medicine. 2014. pp. 341-364

[7] Patil J. Pharmacogenetics and pharmacogenomics: A brief introduction. Journal of Pharmacovigilance. 2015;**2**:3-4

[8] Ma Q, Lu AY. Pharmacogenetics, pharmacogenomics, and individualized medicine. Pharmacological Reviews. 2011;**63**(2):437-459

[9] Xie HG, Frueh FW. Pharmacogenomics steps toward personalized medicine. Future Medicine. 2005:325-337

[10] Crews KR, Hicks JK, Pui CH, Relling MV, Evans WE. Pharmacogenomics and individualized medicine: Translating science into practice. Clinical Pharmacology and Therapeutics. 2012;**92**(4):467-475

[11] Pirmohamed M. Pharmacogenetics and pharmacogenomics. British Journal of Clinical Pharmacology. 2001;**52**(4):345

[12] Tambunan US, Zahroh H, Utomo BB, Parikesit AA. Screening of commercial cyclic peptide as inhibitor NS5 methyltransferase of dengue virus through molecular docking and molecular dynamics simulation. Bioinformation. 2014;**10**(1):23

[13] Tambunan US, Parikesit AA, Prasetia T, Kerami D. In silico molecular interaction studies of suberoylanilide hydroxamic acid and its modified compounds with histones deacetylase class II *Homo sapiens* as curative measure towards cervical cancer. Engineering. 2013;**5**(10):203-206

[14] Parikesit AA. Introductory chapter: The contribution of bioinformatics as blueprint lead for drug design. Molecular Insight of Drug Design. 2018;**29**:7

[15] Handa M, Sharma A, Verma RK, Shukla R. Polycaprolactone based nano-carrier for co-administration of moxifloxacin and rutin and its in-vitro evaluation for sepsis. Journal of Drug Delivery Science and Technology. 2019;**54**:101286

[16] Weinshilboum R, Wang L. Pharmacogenomics: Bench to bedside. Nature Reviews. Drug Discovery. 2004;**3**(9):739-748

[17] Roses AD. Pharmacogenetics and the practice of medicine. Nature. 2000;**405**(6788):857-865

[18] Vizirianakis IS. Challenges in current drug delivery from the potential application of pharmacogenomics and personalized medicine in clinical practice. Current Drug Delivery. 2004;**1**(1):73-80

[19] Kalow W. Pharmacogenetics and pharmacogenomics: Origin, status, and the hope for personalized medicine. The Pharmacogenomics Journal. 2006;**6**(3):162-165

[20] Hicks JK, McLeod HL. Pharmacogenetics and pharmacogenomics. In: Genomic and Precision Medicine. Academic Press; 2017. pp. 89-107

[21] Shastry BS. Pharmacogenetics and the concept of individualized medicine. The Pharmacogenomics Journal. 2006Jan;**6**(1):16-21

[22] Goldstein DB, Tate SK, Sisodiya SM. Pharmacogenetics goes genomic. Nature Reviews. Genetics. 2003;**4**(12):937-947

[23] Valeska MD, Adisurja GP, Bernard S, Wijaya RM, Hafidzhah MA, Parikesit AA. The role of bioinformatics in personalized medicine: Your future medical treatment. Cermin Dunia Kedokteran. 2019;**46**(12):785-788

[24] Agustriawan DA, Sumarpo AN, Parikesit AA, Nurdiansyah RI, Adisurja GP, Putra AR. In silico study of miRNA-regulated IQ motif-containing GTpase-activating protein family in liver cancer. Asian Journal of Pharmaceutical and Clinical Research. 2018;**11**:98-101

[25] National Human Genome Research Institute. All About the Human Genome Project (HGP); 2015

[26] Ikediobi ON, Shin J, Nussbaum RL, Phillips KA, UCSF Center for Translational and Policy Research on Personalized Medicine, Walsh JM, et al. Addressing the challenges of the clinical application of pharmacogenetic testing. Clinical Pharmacology and Therapeutics. 2009;**86**(1):28-31

[27] Kim S, Yun YM, Chae HJ, Cho HJ, Ji M, Kim IS, et al. Clinical pharmacogenetic testing and application: Laboratory medicine clinical practice guidelines. Annals of Laboratory Medicine. 2017;**37**(2):180-193

[28] Voora D, Ginsburg GS. Clinical application of cardiovascular pharmacogenetics. Journal of the American College of Cardiology. 2012;**60**(1):9-20

[29] Ridker PM, Pare G, Parker AN, Zee RY, Miletich JP, Chasman DI. Polymorphism in the CETP gene region, HDL cholesterol, and risk of future myocardial infarction: Genomewide analysis among 18245 initially healthy women from the Women's Genome Health Study. Circulation. Cardiovascular Genetics. 2009;**2**(1):26-33

[30] Anderson CD, Falcone GJ, Phuah CL, Radmanesh F, Brouwers HB, Battey TW, et al. Genetic variants in CETP increase risk of intracerebral hemorrhage. Annals of Neurology. 2016;**80**(5):730-740

[31] Maggo SD, Kennedy MA, Clark DW. Clinical implications of pharmacogenetic variation on the effects of statins. Drug Safety. 2011;**34**(1):1-9

[32] Xiong Z, Ma A, Chen H. JAK3 inhibitors in organ transplantation and autoimmune disease. Recent Patents on Inflammation & Allergy Drug Discovery. 2010;**4**(1):75-81

[33] Säemann MD, Zeyda M, Stulnig TM, Böhmig GA, Wekerle T, Hörl WH, et al. Janus kinase-3 (JAK3) inhibition: a novel immunosuppressive option for

allogeneic transplantation. Transplant International. 2004;**17**(9):481-489

[34] Haan C, Rolvering C, Raulf F, Kapp M, Drückes P, Thoma G, et al. Jak1 has a dominant role over Jak3 in signal transduction through γc-containing cytokine receptors. Chemistry & Biology. 2011;**18**(3):314-323

[35] Spear BB, Heath-Chiozzi M, Huff J. Clinical application of pharmacogenetics. Trends in Molecular Medicine. 2001;**7**(5):201-204

[36] Shah NJ. Regulation of gene expression. In: Introduction to Basics of Pharmacology and Toxicology. Vol. 1: General and Molecular Pharmacology: Principles of Drug Action. 2019. p. 381

[37] Mini E, Nobili S. Pharmacogenetics: Implementing personalized medicine. Clinical Cases in Mineral and Bone Metabolism. 2009;**6**(1):17

[38] Gibbs RA, Belmont JW, Hardenbol P, Willis TD, Yu FL, Yang HM, et al. The international HapMap project. Nature. 2003;**426**(6968):789-796

[39] Manolio TA, Collins FS. The HapMap and genome-wide association studies in diagnosis and therapy. Annual Review of Medicine. 2009;**60**:443-456

[40] Webb A, Hancock JM, Holmes CC. Phylogenetic inference under recombination using Bayesian stochastic topology selection. Bioinformatics. 2009;**25**(2):197-203

[41] Peacock E, Whiteley P. Perlegen sciences, inc. Pharmacogenomics. 2005;**6**(4):439-442

[42] Sachidanandam R, Weissman D, Schmidt SC, Kakol JM, Stein LD, Marth G, et al. A map of human genome sequence variation containing 1.42 million single nucleotide polymorphisms. Nature. 2001;**409**(6822):928-934

[43] Slate J, Gratten J, Beraldi D, Stapley J, Hale M, Pemberton JM. Gene mapping in the wild with SNPs: guidelines and future directions. Genetica. 2009;**136**(1):97-107

[44] Brandl EJ, Kennedy JL, Müller DJ. Pharmacogenetics of antipsychotics. The Canadian Journal of Psychiatry. 2014;**59**(2):76-88

[45] Mallal S, Phillips E, Carosi G, Molina JM, Workman C, Tomažič J, et al. HLA-B* 5701 screening for hypersensitivity to abacavir. The New England Journal of Medicine. 2008;**358**(6):568-579

[46] Weisberg E, Manley PW, Cowan-JacobSW, HochhausA, GriffinJD. Second generation inhibitors of BCR-ABL for the treatment of imatinib-resistant chronic myeloid leukaemia. Nature Reviews. Cancer. 2007;**7**(5):345-356

[47] Dean L. Azathioprine therapy and TPMT and NUDT15 genotype. In: Pratt VM, McLeod HL, Rubinstein WS, et al., editors. Medical Genetics Summaries. Bethesda (MD): National Center for Biotechnology Information (US); 2012

[48] Katz DA, Bhathena A. Overview of pharmacogenetics. Current Protocols in Human Genetics. 2009;**60**(1):9-19

[49] Dervieux T, Bala MV. Overview of the pharmacoeconomics of pharmacogenetics. Future Medicine. 2006;**7**(8):1175-1184

[50] Chouchana L, Narjoz C, Beaune P, Loriot MA, Roblin X. The benefits of pharmacogenetics for improving thiopurine therapy in inflammatory bowel disease. Alimentary Pharmacology & Therapeutics. 2012;**35**(1):15-36

[51] Lin S, Shi Q, Nix FB, Styblo M, Beck MA, Herbin-Davis KM, et al. A novel S-adenosyl-L-methionine: Arsenic (III) methyltransferase from rat liver cytosol. The Journal of Biological Chemistry. 2002;**277**(13):10795-10803

[52] Roje S. S-Adenosyl-L-methionine: Beyond the universal methyl group donor. Phytochemistry. 2006;**67**(15):1686-1698

[53] Chouchana L, Narjoz C, Roche D, Golmard JL, Pineau B, Chatellier G, et al. Interindividual variability in TPMT enzyme activity: 10 years of experience with thiopurine pharmacogenetics and therapeutic drug monitoring. Pharmacogenomics. 2014;**15**(6):745-757

[54] Lennard L. Implementation of TPMT testing. British Journal of Clinical Pharmacology. 2014;**77**(4):704-714

[55] Ford LT, Berg JD. Thiopurine S-methyltransferase (TPMT) assessment prior to starting thiopurine drug treatment; a pharmacogenomic test whose time has come. Journal of Clinical Pathology. 2010;**63**(4):288-295

[56] Moran GW, Dubeau MF, Kaplan GG, Yang H, Eksteen B, Ghosh S, et al. Clinical predictors of thiopurine-related adverse events in Crohn's disease. World Journal of Gastroenterology: WJG. 2015;**21**(25):7795

[57] Roberts RL, Barclay ML. Current relevance of pharmacogenetics in immunomodulation treatment for Crohn's disease. Journal of Gastroenterology and Hepatology. 2012;**27**(10):1546-1554

[58] Wang L, Weinshilboum R. Thiopurine S-methyltransferase pharmacogenetics: insights, challenges and future directions. Oncogene. 2006;**25**(11):1629-1638

[59] Iorio F, Knijnenburg TA, Vis DJ, Bignell GR, Menden MP, Schubert M, et al. A landscape of pharmacogenomic interactions in cancer. Cell. 2016;**166**(3):740-754

[60] Weinstein JN, Collisson EA, Mills GB, Shaw KR, Ozenberger BA, Ellrott K, et al. The cancer genome atlas pan-cancer analysis project. Nature Genetics. 2013;**45**(10):1113

[61] Geeleher P, Zhang Z, Wang F, Gruener RF, Nath A, Morrison G, et al. Discovering novel pharmacogenomic biomarkers by imputing drug response in cancer patients from large genomics studies. Genome Research. 2017;**27**(10):1743-1751

[62] Hughes CA, Foisy MM, Dewhurst N, Higgins N, Robinson L, Kelly DV, et al. Abacavir hypersensitivity reaction: An update. The Annals of Pharmacotherapy. 2008;**42**(3):387-396

[63] Phillips EJ, Chung WH, Mockenhaupt M, Roujeau JC, Mallal SA. Drughypersensitivity:Pharmacogenetics and clinical syndromes. The Journal of Allergy and Clinical Immunology. 2011;**127**(3):S60-S66

[64] Faruki H, Lai-Goldman M. HLA-B* 5701 screening for hypersensitivity to abacavir. Future Medicine. 2008;**5**(3):297-300

[65] Mallal S, Nolan D, Witt C, Masel G, Martin AM, Moore C, et al. Association between presence of HLA-B* 5701, HLA-DR7, and HLA-DQ3 and hypersensitivity to HIV-1 reverse-transcriptase inhibitor abacavir. The Lancet. 2002;**359**(9308):727-732

[66] Mega JL, Stitziel NO, Smith JG, Chasman DI, Caulfield MJ, Devlin JJ, et al. Genetic risk, coronary heart disease events, and the clinical benefit of statin therapy: an analysis of primary and secondary prevention trials. The Lancet. 2015;**385**(9984):2264-2271

[67] Athyros VG, Tziomalos K, Gossios TD, Griva T, Anagnostis P, Kargiotis K, et al. Safety and efficacy of long-term statin treatment for cardiovascular events in patients with coronary heart disease and abnormal liver tests in the Greek Atorvastatin and Coronary Heart Disease Evaluation (GREACE) Study: A post-hoc analysis. The Lancet. 2010;**376**(9756):1916-1922

[68] PEACE Trial Investigators. Angiotensin-converting–enzyme inhibition in stable coronary artery disease. The New England Journal of Medicine. 2004;**351**(20):2058-2068

[69] Santos PC, Krieger JE, Pereira AC. Renin–angiotensin system, hypertension, and chronic kidney disease: Pharmacogenetic implications. Journal of Pharmacological Sciences. 2012;**120**(2):77-88

[70] Trost JC, Lange RA. Treatment of acute coronary syndrome: Part 2: ST-segment elevation myocardial infarction. Critical Care Medicine. 2012;**40**(6):1939-1945

[71] Goedde HW, HW G. Pharmacogenetics of cholinesterase: New variants and suxamethonium sensitivity. Cell Therapy and Gene Therapy. 1979;**25**(9):219-224

[72] Rosenberg H, Pollock N, Schiemann A, Bulger T, Stowell K. Malignant hyperthermia: A review. Orphanet Journal of Rare Diseases. 2015;**10**(1):93

[73] Gätke MR, Bundgaard JR, Viby-Mogensen J. Two novel mutations in the BCHE gene in patients with prolonged duration of action of mivacurium or succinylcholine during anaesthesia. Pharmacogenetics and Genomics. 2007;**17**(11):995-999

[74] Wichmann S, Færk G, Bundgaard JR, Gätke MR. Patients with prolonged effect of succinylcholine or mivacurium had novel mutations in the butyrylcholinesterase gene. Pharmacogenetics and Genomics. 2016;**26**(7):351-356

[75] Daly AK. Pharmacogenetics and human genetic polymorphisms. The Biochemical Journal. 2010;**429**(3):435-449

[76] Zager EM, McNerney R. Multidrug-resistant tuberculosis. BMC Infectious Diseases. 2008;**8**(1):1-5

[77] Warren RM, Streicher EM, van Pittius NG, Marais BJ, Van der Spuy GD, Victor TC, et al. The clinical relevance of mycobacterial pharmacogenetics. Tuberculosis. 2009;**89**(3):199-202

[78] Motta I, Calcagno A, Bonora S. Pharmacokinetics and pharmacogenetics of anti-tubercular drugs: A tool for treatment optimization? Expert Opinion on Drug Metabolism & Toxicology. 2018;**14**(1):59-82

[79] Sim E, Laurieri N. Isoniazid induced toxicity: Systemic lupus erythematosus. Journal of Drug Design and Research. 2018;**49**:51

[80] Rieder MJ, Reiner AP, Gage BF, Nickerson DA, Eby CS, McLeod HL, et al. Effect of VKORC1 haplotypes on transcriptional regulation and warfarin dose. The New England Journal of Medicine. 2005;**352**(22):2285-2293

[81] Johnson JA, Cavallari LH. Warfarin pharmacogenetics. Trends in Cardiovascular Medicine. 2015;**25**(1):33-41

[82] Gulseth MP, Grice GR, Dager WE. Pharmacogenomics of warfarin: Uncovering a piece of the warfarin mystery. American Journal of Health-System Pharmacy. 2009;**66**(2):123-133

[83] Kamali F, Wynne H. Pharmacogenetics of warfarin. Annual Review of Medicine. 2010;**61**:63-75

[84] Limdi NA, Veenstra DL. Warfarin pharmacogenetics. Pharmacotherapy: The Journal of Human Pharmacology and Drug Therapy. 2008;**28**(9):1084-1097

[85] Chasman DI, Ridker PM. Pharmacogenetics: The outlook for genetic testing in statin therapy. Nature Clinical Practice. Cardiovascular Medicine. 2005;**2**(1):2-3

[86] Haase CG, Zuhlsdorf M, Kuhlmann J. The implication of pharmacogenomics/pharmacogenetics on the treatment of neurological diseases. Aktuelle Neurologie. 2002;**29**(7):333-337

[87] Wadelius M, Pirmohamed M. Pharmacogenetics of warfarin: Current status and future challenges. The Pharmacogenomics Journal. 2007;**7**(2):99-111

[88] Li T, Chang CY, Jin DY, Lin PJ, Khvorova A, Stafford DW. Identification of the gene for vitamin K epoxide reductase. Nature. 2004;**427**(6974):541-544

[89] Lurie Y, Loebstein R, Kurnik D, Almog S, Halkin H. Warfarin and vitamin K intake in the era of pharmacogenetics. British Journal of Clinical Pharmacology. 2010;**70**(2):164-170

[90] Dervieux T, Meshkin B, Neri B. Pharmacogenetic testing: Proofs of principle and pharmacoeconomic implications. Mutation Research, Fundamental and Molecular Mechanisms of Mutagenesis. 2005;**573**(1-2):180-194

[91] Vegter S, Boersma C, Rozenbaum M, Wilffert B, Navis G, Postma MJ. Pharmacoeconomic evaluations of pharmacogenetic and genomic screening programmes. PharmacoEconomics. 2008;**26**(7):569-587

Chapter 3

Lipoproteomics: Methodologies and Analysis of Lipoprotein-Associated Proteins along with the Drug Intervention

Julio C. Torres-Romero, Julio César Lara-Riegos, Edgar Antonio Estrella Parra, Verónica Fernández Sánchez, Victor E. Arana-Argáez, Sushally Uc-Colli, Miguel Ángel Peña-Rico, Mario Alberto Ramírez-Camacho, Maria Dolores Ponce Regalado and María Elizbeth Alvarez-Sánchez

Abstract

Lipoproteins are specialized particles involved in the transport and distribution of hydrophobic lipids, as cholesterol and triglycerides, throughout the body. The lipoproteins exhibit a basic spherical shape as complexes of lipids and proteins, and these latter are known as apolipoproteins. Initially, the proteins associated with lipoproteins were recognized as integral or peripheral proteins that only maintain the dynamics and metabolism of lipoproteins. However, there exist many studies on different lipoproteins evidencing that the quantity and type of apolipoproteins and lipoprotein-associated proteins are diverse and could be associated with different lipoprotein function outcomes. Here, we summarized recent processes in the determination of apolipoproteins and lipoprotein-associated proteins profiles through a proteomic approach, analyzing the major methods available and are used to achieve this. We also discuss the relevance of these lipoproteomic analyses on the human disease outcomes.

Keywords: lipoproteins, lipoproteomic, proteomic, high density lipoproteins (HDL), mass spectrometry (MS)

1. Introduction

The emerging high-throughput omics such as genomics, transcriptomics, proteomics, and metabolomics have been used in the search of new biomarkers in several diseases. Proteomic analyses or metabolomics and lipidomics as well as complementary technologies such as mass spectrometry (MS) (i.e., LC-MS-MS and MALDI-TOF/TOF), nuclear magnetic resonance spectroscopy, and other omics technologies, are being widely used in the search of new sources of markers, candidates for vaccine, and alteration of expression patterns in response to environmental changes and signaling pathways in different diseases. The search for proteins in the dynamic system of a proteome requires various proteomics approaches and the use of proteomics is crucial for the early disease diagnosis, prognosis, and to monitor the disease development. The proteomics is essential for the understanding of complex biochemical processes, and the high-throughput proteomics increases the depth of proteome coverage.

Lipoproteins are macromolecular complex particles of lipids and proteins, which are related to the extracellular transport of lipids in many organisms [1]. Besides, lipoproteins have been also implicated as important host defense mediators and in the initiation of immune responses [2–4]. Lipid content has long been recognized as a critical factor in lipoprotein metabolism that acts as an important determinant of human health [5]. However, in last years, apolipoproteins and lipoprotein-associated proteins have been taken on relevance regarding lipoprotein metabolism since they serve as a frame for their assembly, maintain their structure, and interact with the membrane receptors and enzymes. Therefore, these proteins could be crucial in the identification of biomarkers related to diseases due to the fact that they are being studied under a global approach, denominated lipoproteome [6, 7].

2. Lipoprotein structure and metabolism

Lipoproteins are complex protein particles of an amphipathic nature, structurally are formed by an outer layer of phospholipids, free cholesterol, and apolipoproteins, and inside contain a nucleus of cholesterol esters and triglycerides [8]. When the lipoprotein complex is formed, the orientation of the hydrophilic proportions is toward the outside and the lipophilic proportions toward the interior; this structural characteristic allows the complex to have the ability to emulsify fats in extracellular fluids [8]. Based on their density defined by the protein to lipids ratios, lipoproteins are grouped into six classes: chylomicrons, very low density lipoproteins (VLDL), intermediate density lipoproteins (IDL), low density lipoproteins (LDL), high density lipoproteins (HDL), and lipoprotein (a) [Lp (a)] [8, 9].

Triglycerides, derived from dietary fat absorption by the small intestine, are carried by the chylomicrons into blood. After triglyceride digestion to free fatty acids (FFA) by lipases in the peripheral tissues, the size of these particles is reduced, which leads to the formation of chylomicron remnants. These latter are cleared by liver uptake via LDL receptor-related protein (LRP). To synthesize VLDL, newly synthesized triglyceride and cholesterol by the liver are incorporated into chylomicron remnants [8, 10]. These large triglyceride-rich VLDLs are released to the circulation and travel to peripheral tissues, where the lipase digestion of triglycerides occurs resulting in the IDL formation (VLDL remnants). These IDL particles can be either cleared from the circulation by the liver in a similar manner to that described for chylomicrons remnants or can be digested by hepatic lipase to generate cholesterol-rich LDL particles, which is taken up by the peripheral tissues via LDL receptor to supply their cholesterol requirements [10].

The HDL lipoproteins have the highest relative density as compared to other lipoproteins despite being the smallest in size and heterogeneous in terms of composition. These HDL particles play an important role in the transport of reverse cholesterol as a carrier in the movement of cholesterol from peripheral tissues back into the liver [11]. The liver and intestine, practically in response to the lipolysis of triglyceride-rich lipoproteins, synthesize and secrete the nascent discoid HDLs that consist primarily of phospholipids and free cholesterol. Then, these particles reach the plasma where additional exchangeable apolipoproteins are picked up and excess free cholesterol is removed from both extrahepatic cells and other circulating lipoproteins, forming mature spherical HDL particles. Finally, these cholesterol-rich HDL particles can be delivered back to the liver [10, 12].

The protein cargo related to lipoproteins consists of apolipoproteins and lipoprotein-associated proteins. These proteins play key roles in lipoprotein metabolism such as structural component, enzyme interaction, and receptors recognition, among other functions [7]. Changes in the quantity and type of these proteins could be involved in the outcome of diseases related to lipid metabolism. Therefore, the proteomic analysis of lipoproteins is an important notion for the present revision.

3. Apolipoproteins and lipoprotein-associated proteins

The apolipoproteins can be classified as integral or peripheral, either they act as constituent components of the plasma membrane of the lipoproteins or they bind to the membrane and can be exchanged between one complex and another, respectively. Apolipoproteins are distributed throughout all lipoproteins and subfractions, with the proportion of them varying in each family. These variations in the amount of proteins present in the lipoprotein families in their membrane gives them their capacity to interact with different tissues [7, 10].

Within the apolipoprotein A (ApoA) group is the apolipoprotein A-I (ApoA-I), the main protein component of HDL, which plays multiple roles in the transport of cholesterol, in addition to having been linked to the regulation of some functions of the inflammatory and immune response [13]. ApoA-II, also found in HDL, acts as an enzymatic inhibitor of lipoproteins and liver lipases. The apolipoproteins are capable of binding to each other to modify the interaction of the lipoprotein complex, as is the case with apoA-I and apoA-II in LDL [10].

ApoA-IV is mainly synthesized in the small intestine where it is attached by enterocytes to the chylomicrons and secreted during a high-fat meal intake. ApoA-IV is associated with HDL and chylomicron remnants in circulation, but a significant portion is free [14]. On the other hand, ApoA-V participates in the regulation of triglyceride levels in plasma [15]. ApoA-V is expressed only in the liver and circulates at low concentrations. Despite this, apoA-V can be recovered in association with plasma lipoproteins [16].

The apolipoprotein B (ApoB), the main protein component of chylomicrons, LDL, VLDL, IDL, and Lp (a), is encoded by a single gene that gives rises to two isoforms: ApoB-48 and ApoB-100. ApoB-48 is produced exclusively in the intestine and is the major structural protein of chylomicrons and chylomicron remnants. ApoB-100 is expressed in the liver and is found only in VLDL, IDL, LDL, and Lp (a). ApoB-containing lipoproteins are characterized by a spherical shape and contain one single apoB-48 or apoB-100 molecule per lipoprotein [17].

Apolipoprotein C (ApoC) works as an inhibitor of certain processes and modulators of catabolism. ApoC is mainly synthesized in the liver and easily transferred between lipoprotein particles and therefore are found associated with chylomicrons, VLDL, and HDL [10]. ApoC-I is responsible for inhibiting the binding of lipoprotein to its receptor as well as the function of the esterified cholesterol transfer protein (CETP). ApoC-II is an essential cofactor of the lipoprotein lipase involved in triglyceride hydrolysis. Both apoC-III and apoC-IV inhibit triglyceride hydrolysis. In addition, apoC-III decreases the clearance of VLDL [10, 18].

Several tissues synthesize apolipoprotein E (ApoE), an exchangeable apolipoprotein associated with chylomicrons, chylomicron remnants, VLDL, IDL, and a subgroup of HDL particles, but the liver and intestine are the principal producers of circulating ApoE [10]. ApoE functions as a lipoprotein ligator with hepatocytes (clearance of apoE-containing lipoproteins) and peripheral cells related to the LDL receptor. ApoCs and apoEs are interchangeable between complexes during the conversion of VLDL to LDL. ApoEs may function as a lecithin-cholesterol acyltransferase (LCAT) activator and influence the activity of hepatic lipase and CETP [19, 20].

Proteins belonging to the lipocalins family such as apoD, apoM, the orosomucoid protein, and retinol-binding protein (RBP) interact with the surface receptors of the cells, intervening in the formation of macromolecular complexes. It has been described that apoD binds to apoA-II and apoB-100 by means of disulfide bridges; it is associated with LCAT, so it is involved in the transport of lipids in the blood system. ApoJ is involved in a wide variety of processes, acting as a chaperone protein and its main role is the inhibition of lipid transfer and is related to cell death. There are apoproteins such as apoF whose function is unknown; however, there is a theory of their role in abnormal lipid composition inhibiting CETP in the small and dense LDL particles (sdLDL) [21, 22].

In addition to apolipoproteins, lipoproteins require other proteins with specific activities to interact with the environment, which are denominated as lipoprotein-associated proteins. Between these proteins are included phospholipase A2, whose activity indicates the presence of sdLDL in plasma [23]. Serum amyloid A protein (SAA) is associated with several lipoproteins, especially in LDL [24]. Some proteins such as albumin and prenyl cysteine oxidase (PCYOX1) are responsible for protecting against oxidation by lipoproteins such as LDL and splitting the thioether bond of the prenyl cysteine generating H_2O_2, respectively. Also, proteomic studies have identified the apoL-I, PON1, and PAF-AH in small amounts linked to the complexes [25, 26].

The function of many of the proteins that interact with lipoproteins is still unknown. The proteomic analyses have shown that the lipoprotein-associated proteins are involved in cardiovascular risk, immune system, inflammatory processes, among others [7, 26]. However, there is no guide for the analysis of lipoproteins at the proteomic level basically because it depends on the biological question to be investigated, and this determines the approach and the methods or tools to be used as well as the technological platform to perform it.

4. Methodologies used for proteomic analysis of lipoproteins

Before describing the methodologies used for lipoproteomic studies, it is important to mention some general characteristics of lipoprotein-associated proteins and the importance of the research question to establish a good methodological flow chart to address this question. We will start by mentioning that must first consider the lipoprotein obtention by using methods for separation, concentration, and protein stability due to the heterogeneity of these particles.

Diverse chromatographic techniques—prior to proteomic techniques—have been used for the separation of plasma lipoproteins as well as the protein content, such as capillary electrophoresis, size exclusion, cation exchange, gel filtration, fast protein liquid, among other chromatographic techniques [7, 27–32].

The two-dimensional electrophoresis (2-DE) is one of the most usual methods that have been applied to separate the protein cargo related to lipoproteins. Although usually, the first-dimensional separation applied for the proteins in the 2-DE is on base of their charge (isoelectrofocusing), some lipoproteomic analyses have substituted this step by either one of the abovementioned methods to separate lipoproteins or electrophoresis on native gels, followed by SDS-PAGE, which could be denominated as gel-based lipoproteomics [27, 33–35].

Pre-analysis		Chromatography	Mass spectrometry	Analysis	Post-analysis	
Source	**Methods**	**chromatographic technique = Instrumentation (method)**	**Mass analyzer = Instrumentation (method)**	**Database search**	**Number of lipoproteins and apoproteins**	**References**
Mice C57BL/6 J: plasma	Gel filtration/size exclusion chromatography, phospholipid-containing particles using CSH	LC-ESI = C_{18} reverse phase column (GRACE; 150 × 0.500 mm)	Quadrupole/TOF = 4800 scans, mass range: 300–1800 *m/z*, charge states:2–5, excluded target ions: 300 s	Swiss-Prot protein knowledge base for *Mus musculus*, PeptideProphet algorithm	VLDL/LDL: 32, HDL: 104; lipid poor lipoproteins: 55	[37]
Human serum (HDL)	Trypsin, delipidation, gold nanoparticles and LDI-MS, EDX, SPE, FT-IR		MALDI-MS = nr	Swiss-Prot, Lipidmaps database	HDL (delipidation): 10 (prior), 6 (after). HDL (anion exchangers): 23	[38]
Mice C57BL/6 J: apoA-I KO and apoA-II KO, apoA-I KO and WT: plasma	Particles of CSH. Plasma separation by size exclusion chromatography	LC-ESI = column (C18 reverse phase (150 × 0.500 mm))	Quadrupole/TOF = MS/MS. tolerance were set to ±35 PPM, and up to 3 missed tryptic cleavage sites were allowed	UniProtKB/Swiss-Prot Protein Knowledgebase, Peptide Prophet algorithm	HDL: WT:25 vs. ApoA-I KO: 21; ApoA-II KO: 11 vs. WT: 14; and ApoA-IV: 6 KO vs. WT: 7	[28]
17 Subjects (exposure to organic pollutants): plasma (HDL)	Ultracentrifugation (290,000 g, 15°C, 4 h)	nLC: Column C18, ESI	Linear ion trap-Orbitrap: CID. ms/ms: 0.6 Da	MaxQuant v1.5.0, human Uniprot/Swiss-prot database	LCMS permit identified the pathway of interaction between HDL-proteins	[39]
34 Men (2 dietary: weight loss/high car): plasma (LDL, ApoC-III)	ELISA assay		MALDI-TOF: 500 laser shots mass spectra		Detection and concentrations values of 12 apoC-III glycoforms	[40]
Mice (female, LDLr−/−, 8 week old): plasma (VLDL, LDL, HDL)	FPLC, ELISA assay	LC	Orbitrap: mass tolerance: 0.8 Da	Swiss-Prot database	HDL: 91 LDL: 49 VLDL: 39	[41]
1000 Children (6–8 years, Nepal rural zone): plasma	Cation exchange chromatography	LC	Orbitrap	Refseq 40 database	Apo-AI, Apo-AII, Apo-CIII	[42]

Pre-analysis		Chromatography	Mass spectrometry	Analysis	Post-analysis	
Source	**Methods**	**chromatographic technique = Instrumentation (method)**	**Mass analyzer = Instrumentation (method)**	**Database search**	**Number of lipoproteins and apoproteins**	**References**
458 Children (6–11 years, exposure to environmental tobacco smoke): serum (HDL, LDL)		SPE-HPLC-TIS-MS/MS			LC detected various polyfluoroalkyl substances in serum A negative association PFOS and non-HDL	[43]
57 Males (exposed to arsenicum): plasma, urinary (LDL, HDL, Lp(a), Apo-A1, Apo-B)	Centrifuged at 3500 rpm for 10 min		ICP-MS: extraction voltage −100 V, Rf power 1400 W, focus voltage 12 V, and nebulizer gas flow rate (using a Burgener Miramist nebulizer) 0.83 L/min. Dwell times were 50 ms for 75As and 10 ms for internal standard (72 Ge)		ICP-MS: Potential risk of the arsenic on lipoproteins and apolipoproteins	[44]
Human healthy, normolipidemic males: plasma (LDL)	Gel filtration chromatography, ultracentrifugation.	nLC: column (IntePepMap 100, C18, particle size 3 um), flow rate = 300 nL/min ESI: 2.5 kV, 150°C	Triple quadrupole TOF: mass tolerance: 50 mDa, 350–1800 *m/z* window, MSscan type: 0.25 s	UniProtKB/Swiss-Prot Protein Knowledgebase, Peptide Prophet algorithm	LC-MS permit the abundance protein as well as antioxidant activity	[30]
110 Samples (purchased)		Phospholipids: UHPLC: column (2.1 × 100 mm, 1.7 uM particle), flow rate: 0.7 mL/min, ESI	Qtrap: MRM scanning, negative and positive mode	Multiquant software functions, JMP (SAS Institute)	LC-MS analysis of serum/lipoproteins	[45]
23 Healthy volunteers: serum	Gel filtration chromatography, sequential ultracentrifugation, immunoassay	UPLC: column (UPLCR BEH C8), floe rate: 450 uL/min., 60°C, autosampler: 4°C ESI	Triple-quadrupole: positive ion mode. Quantification of plasmalogens: Capillary voltage: 3500 V, source temperature 80°C, desolvation: 400°C, cone voltage: 35 V. CE: 20–32 eV		LCMS: distribution of each molecular species in plasmalogen and choline plasmalogen	[46]

Pre-analysis		Chromatography	Mass spectrometry	Analysis	Post-analysis	
Source	Methods	chromatographic technique = Instrumentation (method)	Mass analyzer = Instrumentation (method)	Database search	Number of lipoproteins and apoproteins	References
Healthy volunteers: plasma (VLDL, LDL, HDL)	Ultracentrifugation, SDS-PAGE, size exclusion chromatography, circular dichroism, spectroscopy, spectropolarimeter		MALDI-TOF: 337 nm nitrogen laser, positive ion: 20 kV		Identification of apolipoproteins released from VLDL by mass spectrometry	[47]
20 Patients with lipoproteins (a) (18–70 years): plasma (LDL, HDL)	Ultracentrifugation, ELISA	LC: solid-phase extraction	Triple Quadrupole-linear ion tramp: SRM. (energy collision: 34 V, Q1: 786–788; Q2: 1069–1072 *m/z*)		LC-MS system: concentrations of lipid, lipoprotein and apolipoprotein	[48]
Healthy donors (nonlipidemic, 24–65 years, purchased samples): plasma (HDL, LDL)	Ultracentrifugation (330,000 g, 6 h), SDS-PAGE and Western blotting, Negative stain electron microscopy	UPLC: column (Kinetex EVOC18), ESI	Triple-quadrupole: lipid species were analyzed by selected reaction monitoring (from 141 to 369 *m/z*, from 0 to 50 eV)	Extraction and ionization efficacy by calculating analyte/ISTD ratios (AU) and expressed as AU/mg protein	LCS permit the separation of a mixture in HDL protein	[49]
12 Healthy male (36–67 years): plasma (HDL, LDL)	Ultracentrifugation (40,000 rpm, 44 h, 15°C), fractioned, apoA-I was detected by Western blotting, internal standars	HILIC-UHPLC-FLD: Glycan chromatography column, 150 × 2.1 mm i.d., 1.7 μm BEH particles, flow rate of 0.56 mL/min	MALDI-TOF-MS: 25 kV, acceleration voltage: 140 ns extraction delay, mass window: 1000–5000 *m/z*. For each spectrum: 10,000 laser shots, laser frequency of 2000 Hz		LDL: 18 HDL: 22 N-glycome of human plasma lipoproteins	[50]
16 Healthy adults: plasma (HDL, apoA-I, apoB)	Ultracentrifugation. PRM analysis (shotgun proteomics experiments).	UPLC: flow rate: 0.6 uL, column (Xbridge BEH C18) ESI	Orbitrap: PRM mode, isolation window: 2 Th, HCD: 27%, orbitrap analyzer: 15,000 resolution, AGC: 5 × 10^4, maximum ion time 30 ms	PeptideAtlas mass spectral database	Meal macronutrient content HDL composition in the postprandial state	[51]

Pre-analysis		Chromatography	Mass spectrometry	Analysis	Post-analysis	
Source	**Methods**	**chromatographic technique = Instrumentation (method)**	**Mass analyzer = Instrumentation (method)**	**Database search**	**Number of lipoproteins and apoproteins**	**References**
47 Volunteers: serum (HDL, non-HDL).	Anti-apoAI magnetic nanoparticles (10 mg) and serum (5 µl) were mixed FTIR, X-ray diffraction	ID/LC/MS system: LC: column (waters symmetry C18), flow rate: 0.3 mL/min. APCI: corona current: 5 uA, source temperature: 450°C	API 4000 tandem mass spectrometer (triple-quadrupole): Collision energy: 26 eV, collision exit potential: 6 V		ID/LC-MS permit the monitoring serum in clinical settings to dyslipidemia and atherosclerosis	[52]

SRM: selected reaction monitoring. HPLC: high performance liquid chromatography. HILIC-UHPLC-FLD: hydrophilic-interaction ultra-high-performance liquid chromatography with fluorescence detection. LC: liquid Chromatography. UPLC: ultra-performance liquid chromatography. MALDI: matrix-assisted laser desorption/ionization. TOF: time of flight. Qtrap or LTQ linear trap: triple quadrupole-linear ion trap. CE: collision energy. MS/MS: tandem mass spectrometry. PRM: parallel reaction monitoring. AGC: automatic gain control. ID/LC/MS: isotope dilution liquid chromatography mass spectrometry. ESI: electrospray. nESI: nano-electrospray. FPLC: fast protein liquid chromatography. MRM: multiple reaction monitoring. HILIC: silica-based and solid-core reverse phase after hydrophilic interaction. ICP-MS: Inductively coupled plasma-mass spectrometer. SPE: solid phase extraction. SPE-HPLC-TIS-MS/MS: solid phase extraction coupled to high performance liquid chromatography-turbo ion spray ionization-tandem mass spectrometry. SEC-FPLC: size exclusion chromatography by fast protein liquid chromatography. APCI: atmospheric pressure chemical ionization. CID: collision-induced dissociation. LDI-MS: laser desorption/ionization mass spectrometry, EDX: dispersive X-Ray Spectroscopy. CSH: calcium silica hydrate. WT: wild-type. KO: knockout. FTIR: Fourier transformation infrared.

Table 1.
Chromatographic and spectrometric methodologies used recently in lipoproteomic analysis.

Pre-analysis |		Spectroscopy experiment NMR type	Post-analysis	References
Source	isolation method			
133 Caucasian participants (T2DM, >18 years): serum (VLDL, LDL, and HDL)		1H: FT, 400 MHz	Determinate the lipoprotein subtraction characteristics	[56]
98 people (T2DM/ nor T2DM): plasma (GlycA vs. Lp-PLA2)	Centrifugation (1400 g, 15 min)	^{1}H: 400 MHz, 47° C, CaEDTA resonance at 2.519 ppm was used as the internal chemical	GlycA is correlated with LP-PLA2 in plasma (person without T2DM/ MetS)	[57]
23 patients with primary aldosteronism: plasma (HDL, VLDL, LDL, ApoB, and ApoA-I)	Immunoturbidimetric assay	^{1}H: 400 MHz, 47° C. (LipoProfile-3 algorithm)	Circulating LDL may contribute to adrenal steroidogenesis in humans	[58]
115 nondiabetic women (35–55 years, mediterranean diet, physical exercise, 2 years): plasma (HDL. LDL)		^{1}H	Lipoprotein size, particle and subclass concentrations	[54]
Human serum (purchased) spiked into phlebotomy tubes (LDL, HDL)	Centrifugation (3000 g, 5 min, 4 h)	^{1}H: 600 MHz	Lipoprotein subclass analysis standardized by tube type and tube size to prevent risk of analytical interference.	[59]
Patients with HFrEF (782), HFpEF (1004), and no HF (4742): plasma (HDL)		NMR LipoProfile-3 algorithm	Quantify concentrations of HDL. Phenotyped cohorts of HFrEF, HFpEF, and patients without HF	[60]
4897 subjects: plasma (LDL)		^{1}H: 400 MHz	Differentiate in the size of particle in LDL profile	[61]
309 patients (MACE): plasma (HDL, LDL, and VLDL). Control:902		^{1}H	Neither baseline HDL nor the change in HDL on treatment with dalcetrapib or placebo was associated with risk of MACE after ACS	[62]
Normal volunteer: plasma (HDL, LDL, andVLDL)	Sequential ultracentrifuge	1H, ^{13}C, ^{15}N: 600.55 MHz, 47° C, different pressures	Show the spatial arrangement, phase behavior and molecular dynamics in the particle core	[55]
3446 participants (HDL, LDL, and VLDL)		^{1}H: LipoProfile-3 algorithm	Association between FGF21 and NAFLD	[63]

MHz: megahertz (10^6). MetS or MS: metabolic syndrome. T2DM: type 2 Diabetes mellitus. FT: Fourier transforms. CaEDTA: EDTA mono calcium. GlycA: glycoprotein acetylation. Lp-PLA2: lipoprotein-associated phospholipase A2. HFrEF: reduced ejection fractions. HFpEF: preserved ejection fraction. HF: heart failure. MACE: major adverse cardiovascular events. FGF21: fibroplast growth factor21. NAFLD: nonalcoholic fatty liver disease.

Table 2.
NMR methodology applied recently in lipoprotein-based analyses.

Lipoprotein-associated proteins are not easy to study by proteomic methods, mainly the embedded in the lipoprotein membranes. These latter have rigid transmembrane domains that contain α-helices or β-barrels, which stabilize the protein by strong secondary structural characteristics and these regions can resist proteolytic digestion [6, 36]. Thus, the protein identification for lipoproteomes has been mainly performed by two methods: mass spectrometry and resonance magnetic nuclear.

Modern mass spectrometry (MS) techniques have allowed for thorough characterizations of the lipoproteins [37]. However, different experimental conditions have been reported to avoid contamination of the biological samples as well as selective and optimized methods to detect lipoproteins, usually liquid-phase separation techniques, prior to spectrometric techniques [36, 37]. Thus, different spectrometric experimentation conditions have been reported for the study of lipoproteins and apoproteins, respectively (**Table 1**).

There are several challenges in the lipoproteomic analyses performed with the most advanced mass spectrometry methods. Some of them are the abundance of proteins from the biological source and the lipoprotein(s) purification steps, which conditioned the protein content and constitution. However, if this obstacle can be overcome, the mass spectrometry analysis has been demonstrated to be a useful tool to identify a diverse array of proteins related to lipoproteins, avoiding aberrant integration of unexpected proteins by reducing the suppression of ionization at high peptide resolution [53].

On the other hand, the nuclear magnetic resonance (NMR) technique permit, besides protein identification, can provide information of the lipoproteins at both molecule and atomic levels under physiological or 'near-physiological' conditions. The signal most used to quantify lipoproteins is the methyl signal because give a specific response in the lipids that travel inside the lipoproteins [54, 55]. In this way, proton spectroscopy has been the most used nuclear magnetic resonance technique to quantify lipoproteins, but it is not the only one as will be seen later (**Table 2**).

Furthermore, not only ^{1}H NMR has been the technique used for the study of lipoproteomics but also the two-dimensional NMR techniques have been used. The two-dimensional heteronuclear $^{13}C—^{1}H$ chemical-shift made it possible to analyze macromolecular complexes like HDL, but with a limited resolution in reduced peaks above 50 ppm and the limited resolution in the 29–33 ppm region, inclusive with artifacts that would later be discarded by the spectra of one dimension (^{1}H and ^{13}C) [64].

In addition, the material to be used for the spectroscopic analysis should be the optimal one to avoid contamination, as in the case of a tube used for the collection of biological material and used in clinical research, which should be specifically for the analysis of lipoproteins [59].

Also, the experimental conditions do not always favor the use of NMR for the analysis of lipoproteins. Thus, mass spectrometry permits the particle identification via LC-MS system in contrast to NMR spectroscopy, which failed. Due to that, the NMR spectroscopy makes HDL particle quantification only in a physiological setting: full serum or plasma but not in HDL-containing suspensions [49]. Therefore, the technician must consider the biological and technical variables for an assertive lipoproteomic analysis.

5. Clinical significance of lipoproteomic analyses

The lipoproteomic analyses have been focused on understanding the functional mechanisms underlying apolipoproteins and lipoprotein-associated proteins that can be used to develop new diagnostic and/or prognostic biomarkers for many lipoproteins' metabolism-related illness.

The HDL lipoprotein fraction has been the most studied according to lipoproteomic relationships with different diseases. Among the HDL-associated proteins, ApoC-III levels have been seen increased in the patients with either a lupus nephritis (lupus erythematosus) or with a cerebral lacunar infarction, which could be related with a reduced anti-inflammatory activity of HDL particles [65, 66].

However, HDL-carried ApoC-III has been more implicated in cardiovascular disease (CVD) risk. One of the first evaluations was performed with coronary artery disease patients, which exhibit increased levels of ApoC-III [67]. Recently, in a cohort study, it was demonstrated that HDL-carried ApoC-III is related to a higher risk for coronary heart disease [68].

In addition to ApoC-III and ApoC-II, other HDL-associated apolipoproteins, were proposed as biomarkers for CVD risk in patients with chronic hemodialysis [69]. The ApoC-III/ApoC-II/ApoE levels in VLDL lipoproteins, independent of HDL, were associated with incident CVD, which supports the concept of targeting triacylglycerol-rich lipoproteins to reduce the CVD risk [70].

Other HDL-associated apolipoproteins have been associated with cardiac pathologies. For example, ApoA-I, ApoA-IV, ApoE, and ApoL1 levels have been seen enriched in HDL3 fraction from patients with acute coronary syndrome (ACV), with a concomitant reduction of these apolipoproteins in the HDL2 fraction [71]. Furthermore, ApoC-I was significantly decreased in the HDL particles of coronary heart disease (CAD) patients in comparison to normal individuals [72]. The existence of CAD has recently been correlated with an HDL apolipoproteomic score, independent of circulating ApoA-I and ApoB rates and other typical cardiovascular risk factors [73].

Regarding HDL-associated proteins, many of them have been related to heart illness. For example, serotransferrin, haptoglobin, hemopexin, complement factor B, ras-related protein Rab-7b, and paraoxonase-3 (PON3) levels have been seen reduced in HDL from patients with some cardiac pathology. Meanwhile, PON1, alpha-1B-glycoprotein, vitamin D-binding protein, alpha-1-antitrypsin (A1AT), acid ceramidase, serum amyloid A and P proteins, sphingosine-1-phosphate, filamin A, and pulmonary surfactant-associated protein B are increased in HDL fractions from patients with cardiometabolic disorders [69, 71, 72, 74, 75].

Diabetes is, perhaps, the major controllable risk factor for CVD. In particular, related to the HDL fraction, ApoA-I, ApoA-II, ApoA-IV, ApoE, ApoJ, as well as PON1, transthyretin, complement C3, and vitamin D-binding protein have shown changes in patients with type 2 diabetes (T2D) [76, 77]. In contrast, individuals with type 1 diabetes (T1D) had proteomic alterations of their HDL particles. For example, the complement factor H-related protein 2 was elevated, independent of glucose control, in T1D patients in comparison to healthy controls. Also, the optimal glucose control corrected the elevated levels of the alpha-1-beta glycoprotein and inter alpha trypsin inhibitor 4. Furthermore, the HDL particles in T1DM individuals, independent of glucose control, exhibit a higher abundance of irreversible post-translational modifications of HDL-associated apolipoproteins [78, 79].

Also, in psoriatic patients, the levels of HDL-associated ApoA-I exhibit a significant reduction, whereas levels of apoA-II, serum amyloid A, C3, and A1AT, among other proteins were increased [80]. Besides C3 and C9, complement factor B, as well as ApoJ, fibrinogen, haptoglobin, and serum amyloid A have been also increased in HDL fraction from patients with rheumatoid arthritis [81]. Taken together, these results suggest that HDL-associated proteins could be involved in anti-inflammatory properties in chronic illness.

Concerning other diseases, the proteome of HDL particles has been used to identify protein markers. In nonalcoholic fatty liver disease, including individuals with nonalcoholic steatohepatitis, changes in the abundance of HDL-associated proteins such as antithrombin III and plasminogen have been identified [82]. Although not directly to HDL particles, proteomic analysis of some HDL-related apolipoproteins has been associated with viral diseases. For example, a change in the expression level of ApoA-I was suggested as a specific and appropriate alternative to conventional HIV diagnosis and progression measurements in clinical research settings [83]. Increased concentration of ApoM in sera patients with HBV infection have been detected [84]. Recently, a downregulation of ApoA-I and ApoM levels have been associated with the severity of COVID-19 infection [85].

In addition to HDL, only other few lipoproteomic studies have been developed to discover changes in lipoproteins-associated proteins in diverse pathologies. Proteomic studies of LDL have reported that carry apolipoproteins AI, A-II, CI, C-II, C-III, C-IV, D, E, and F, in addition to apoB, as well as clusterin, C3, C4a, and C4b, and PON1 that are also associated to this particles [86]. Serum amyloid A levels were found to increase in all lipoprotein fractions, especially in LDL from atherosclerotic patients [24]. An enriched content of all the apoC-III isoforms and a lower content of apoA-I, apoC-I, and apoE were detected in the sdLDL from subjects with metabolic syndrome and subclinical peripheral atherosclerosis [87]. VLDL, IDL, and LDL fractions from Alzheimer patients exhibit low levels of complement C3 [88].

6. HDL lipoproteomics for drug discovery

Target discovery, which is an important step in the drug development process, includes discovering and validating targets associated with the diseases. It is increasingly recognized that, in many instances, metabolomics is used to identify novel biomarkers, which can help in the discovery of therapeutic strategies for many diseases [89].

Until now, lipoproteomics has proved to be an effective method for identifying candidate cardiovascular disease markers. Studying the profiles of protein expression in drug-treated patients contributes to the discovery of multiple drug-specific targets. Traditionally, statin therapy has proven efficacy in reducing cardiovascular events, but as aforementioned, the identification of HDL-associated proteins is variable. The statin therapy has a notorious effect on the increment of A1AT associated to the large fraction of HDL particles enhancing its anti-inflammatory functionality, which may interfere with the statins outcome on reducing cholesterol levels [37]. In addition, a relationship between the CAD treatment and the HDL proteome was demonstrated using statin and niacin therapy, observing that ApoE and ApoC-II levels are enriched in the HDL3 fraction, which contains less ApoJ levels [90].

The increment in the HDL levels by CETP inhibitors is another biomarker that has continued to be disappointing in clinical research. In fact, in patients with deficiency of CETP (CETP-D), the HDL particles are enriched with ApoE, angiopoietin-like3 protein, and complement regulatory proteins such as C3, C4a, C4b, and C9 that could be associated to the increased atherogenic profile in CETP-D patients [91].

Thus, it is important to consider that among the diverse HDL populations not all possess a cardioprotective effect [92]. Therefore, we need a better knowledge of the protein cargo of the HDL populations with anti-atherogenic actions. A comprehensive understanding of the HDL proteomics can lead to the design of more effective anti-atherogenic drugs based on the activity of HDL-associated proteins that will provide new therapeutic strategies at the molecular level.

In the dynamic drug discovery process, the different proteomic methods, which include MS-proteomics, expand beyond the general aim of target drug discovery. It must consider the drug-protein interactions as well as elucidate the mode of action of candidate drug molecules [93]. Thus, novel HDL-based therapeutic agents, besides the traditional statins, will need consider to the functional HDL lipoproteomics to characterize the interaction of the drug with the HDL-associated proteins. This is necessary as an attempt either to elucidate the mechanism of action by direct drug-protein interaction or as a biomarker for drug validation by monitoring the pharmacological effect through an increase of HDL populations with an anti-atherogenic protein cargo.

7. Conclusion

The lipoproteins can be involved in different pathologies related to lipid metabolism such as atherosclerosis, cardiovascular risk, obesity, metabolic síndrome, and diabetes, among others. However, the protein cargo of these particles has been associated with several functions, which differ from the amply recognized as structural composition and receptors recognition during their function as lipid transporters. For this reason, the identification of variants of apolipoproteins and lipoprotein-associated proteins has been an important referent to detect new biomarkers. In fact, as we described here, several methodologies have been developed to improve the lipoproteomic profile.

Despite these studies, the majority concord that both biological source and lipoprotein purification are important steps to avoid protein contamination, principally from samples that are used directly as serum or plasma. Also, the most used method to identify the lipoprotein-associated proteins is the mass spectrometry, but some limits are presented that depend on the platforms to apply this methodology. Also, it is important to highlight that not everyone has the facility to use this methodology and it is necessary to develop new methodologies to apply in clinical fields to ensure discoveries about these proteins both in new lipoproteins' fractions and new diseases.

Also, the lipoproteomic analyses could be a new clinical area to evaluate the therapy of the pathologies described here as prognostic analytes. In this sense, the HDL lipoproteomics is, perhaps, the more advanced field considering the evaluations of populations with statins' treatment. However, novel HDL therapeutic agents must consider the functional lipoproteomics of these particles. Finally, these lipoproteomes can help us to describe the molecular mechanism to understand the interaction of apolipoproteins as well as the lipoprotein-carried proteins to support the other omics such as lipidomics and metabolomics.

Acknowledgements

This work was supported by the Autonomous University of Mexico City (UACM) awarded to MEAS.

Conflict of interest

The authors declare no conflict of interest.

Author details

Julio C. Torres-Romero[1†], Julio César Lara-Riegos[1†], Edgar Antonio Estrella Parra[2], Verónica Fernández Sánchez[3], Victor E. Arana-Argáez[1], Sushally Uc-Colli[1], Miguel Ángel Peña-Rico[4], Mario Alberto Ramírez-Camacho[1], Maria Dolores Ponce Regalado[5] and María Elizbeth Alvarez-Sánchez[6*]

1 Chemistry Faculty, Autonomous University of Yucatán (UADY), Merida, Mexico

2 Laboratory of Phytochemistry, UBIPRO, National Autonomous University of Mexico, Mexico City, Mexico

3 Faculty of Higher Studies (FES), National Autonomous University of Mexico, Mexico City, Mexico

4 Institute of Biotechnology, University of Papaloapan, Oaxaca, Mexico

5 Department of Health Sciences, Los Altos University of Guadalajara, Mexico

6 Genomic Sciences Postgraduate, Autonomous University of Mexico City (UACM), Mexico City, Mexico

*Address all correspondence to: maria.alvarez@uacm.edu.mx; elizbeth2@gmail.com

[†]Co-first authors.

References

[1] Pan L, Segrest JP. Computational studies of plasma lipoprotein lipids. Biochimica et Biophysica Acta (BBA) - Biomembranes. 2016;**1858**(10): 2401-2420

[2] Han R. Plasma lipoproteins are important components of the immune system. Microbiology and Immunology. 2010;**54**(4):246-253

[3] Kaji H. High-density lipoproteins and the immune system. Journal of Lipids. 2013;**2013**:684903

[4] Bora K, Borah P. Plasma lipoproteins as crucial components of host defence against infections. In: Isbir T, editor. Advances in Lipoprotein Research. London, UK: IntechOpen; 2017. pp. 73-92. DOI: 10.5772/67601

[5] Ogedegbe HO, Brown DW. Lipids, lipoproteins, and apolipoproteins and their disease associations. Laboratory Medicine. 2001;**32**(7):384-389

[6] Hoofnagle AN, Heinecke JW. Lipoproteomics: Using mass spectrometry-based proteomics to explore the assembly, structure, and function of lipoproteins. Journal of Lipid Research. 2009;**50**(10):1967-1975

[7] von Zychlinski A, Kleffmann T. Dissecting the proteome of lipoproteins: New biomarkers for cardiovascular diseases? Translational Proteomics. 2015;7:30-39

[8] Jovandaric MZ, Milenkovic SJ. Significance of lipid and lipoprotein in organism. In: Lipoproteins and Apolipoproteins-New Perspectives and Applications. London, UK: IntechOpen; 2020. DOI: 10.5772/intechopen.91407

[9] Jawi MM, Frohlich J, Chan SY. Lipoprotein (a) the insurgent: A new insight into the structure, function, metabolism, pathogenicity, and medications affecting lipoprotein (a) molecule. Journal of Lipids. 2020; **2020**:3491764. DOI: 10.1155/2020/3491764

[10] Feingold KR, Grunfeld C. Introduction to lipids and lipoproteins. In: Endotext [Internet]. Dartmouth, Massachusetts, USA: MDText.com, Inc.; 2018

[11] Zhou L, Li C, Gao L, Wang A. High-density lipoprotein synthesis and metabolism. Molecular Medicine Reports. 2015;**12**(3):4015-4021

[12] Trajkovska KT, Topuzovska S. High-density lipoprotein metabolism and reverse cholesterol transport: Strategies for raising HDL cholesterol. Anatolian Journal of Cardiology. 2017; **18**(2):149-154

[13] Georgila K, Vyrla D, Drakos E. Apolipoprotein AI (ApoA-I), immunity, inflammation and cancer. Cancers. 2019;**11**(8):1097

[14] Wang F, Kohan AB, Lo CM, Liu M, Howles P, Tso P. Thematic review series: Intestinal lipid metabolism: New developments and current insights: Apolipoprotein A-IV: A protein intimately involved in metabolism. Journal of Lipid Research. 2015;**56**(8): 1403-1418

[15] Pennacchio LA, Olivier M, Hubacek JA, et al. An apolipoprotein influencing triglycerides in humans and mice revealed by comparative sequencing. Science. 2001;**294**(5540): 169-173

[16] Gonzales JC, Gordts PLSM, Foley EM, et al. Apolipoproteins E and AV mediate lipoprotein clearance by hepatic proteoglycans. The Journal of Clinical Investigation. 2013;**123**(6): 2742-2751

[17] Sniderman AD, Thanassoulis G, Glavinovic T, Navar AM, Pencina M, Catapano A, et al. Apolipoprotein B particles and cardiovascular disease: A narrative review. JAMA Cardiology. 2019;**4**(12):1287-1295

[18] Jin JL, Guo YL, Li JJ. Apoprotein C-III: A review of its clinical implications. Clinica Chimica Acta. 2016;**460**:50-54

[19] Getz GS, Reardon CA. Apoprotein E and reverse cholesterol transport. International Journal of Molecular Sciences. 2018;**19**(11):3479. DOI: 10.3390/ijms19113479

[20] Amaya-Montoya M, Pinzón-Cortés JA, Silva-Bermúdez LS, Ruiz-Manco D, Pérez-Matos MC, Jiménez-Mora MA, et al. ApoE and apoC-III-defined HDL subtypes: A descriptive study of their lecithin cholesterol acyl transferase and cholesteryl ester transfer protein content and activity. Lipids in Health and Disease. 2020;**19**(1):1-11

[21] Davidson WS, Silva RGD, Chantepie S, Lagor WR, Chapman MJ, Kontush A. Proteomic analysis of defined HDL subpopulations reveals particle-specific protein clusters: Relevance to antioxidative function. Arteriosclerosis, Thrombosis, and Vascular Biology. 2009;**29**(6):870-876

[22] Kontush A, Lindahl M, Lhomme M, Calabresi L, Chapman MJ, Davidson WS. Structure of HDL: Particle subclasses and molecular components. In: High Density Lipoproteins. Cham: Springer; 2015. pp. 3-51

[23] Gazi I, Lourida ES, Filippatos T, Tsimihodimos V, Elisaf M, Tselepis AD. Lipoprotein-associated phospholipase A2 activity is a marker of small, dense LDL particles in human plasma. Clinical Chemistry. 2005;**51**(12):2264-2273

[24] Lepedda AJ, Nieddu G, Zinellu E, De Muro P, Piredda F, Guarino A, et al. Proteomic analysis of plasma-purified VLDL, LDL, and HDL fractions from atherosclerotic patients undergoing carotid endarterectomy: Identification of serum amyloid A as a potential marker. Oxidative Medicine and Cellular Longevity. 2013. DOI: 10.1155/2013/385214

[25] Sun HY, Chen SF, Lai MD, Chang TT, Chen TL, Li PY, et al. Comparative proteomic profiling of plasma very-low-density and low-density lipoproteins. Clinica Chimica Acta. 2010;**411**(5–6):336-344

[26] Baig F, Joshi A, Mayr M. High-density lipoproteins in high resolution: Will proteomics solve the paradox for cardiovascular risk? Proteomics. 2017;**17** (3–4). DOI: 10.1002/pmic.201600426

[27] Karlsson H, Leanderson P, Tagesson C, Lindahl M. Lipoproteomics I: Mapping of proteins in low-density lipoprotein using two-dimensional gel electrophoresis and mass spectrometry. Proteomics. 2005;**5**(2):551-565

[28] Gordon SM, Li H, Zhu X, Tso P, Reardon CA, Shah AS, et al. Impact of genetic deletion of platform apolipoproteins on the size distribution of the murine lipoproteome. Journal of Proteomics. 2016;**146**:184-194

[29] Huang LH, Zinselmeyer BH, Chang CH, Saunders BT, Elvington A, Baba O, et al. Interleukin-17 drives interstitial entrapment of tissue lipoproteins in experimental psoriasis. Cell Metabolism. 2018;**9**(2):475-487

[30] Swertfeger DK, Rebholz S, Li H, Shah AS, Davidson WS, Lu LJ. Feasibility of a plasma bioassay to assess oxidative protection of low-density lipoproteins by high-density lipoproteins. Journal of Clinical Lipidology. 2018;**12**(6):1539-1548

[31] Phipps ZC, Seck F, Davis AN, Rico JE, McFadden JW. Characterization of ceramide in bovine

lipoproteins. Journal of Dairy Science. 2017;**100**(10):8602-8608

[32] Olkowicz M, Debski J, Jablonska P, Dadlez M, Smolenski RT. Application of a new procedure for liquid chromatography/mass spectrometry profiling of plasma amino acid-related metabolites and untargeted shotgun proteomics to identify mechanisms and biomarkers of calcific aortic stenosis. Journal of Chromatography A. 2017; **1517**:66-78

[33] Mancone C, Amicone L, Fimia GM, Bravo E, Piacentini M, Tripodi M, et al. Proteomic analysis of human very low-density lipoprotein by two-dimensional gel electrophoresis and MALDI-TOF/TOF. Proteomics. 2007;**7**(1):143-154

[34] Bancells C, Canals F, Benítez S, Colomé N, Julve J, Ordóñez-Llanos J, et al. Proteomic analysis of electronegative low-density lipoprotein. Journal of Lipid Research. 2010;**51**(12):3508-3515

[35] Holzer M, Kern S, Birner-Grünberger R, Curcic S, Heinemann A, Marsche G. Refined purification strategy for reliable proteomic profiling of HDL 2/3. Impact on proteomic complexity. Scientific Reports. 2016;**6**(1):1-10

[36] Vaisar T. Thematic review series: Proteomics. Proteomic analysis of lipid-protein complexes. Journal of Lipid Research. 2009;**50**(5):781-786

[37] Gordon SM, McKenzie B, Kemeh G, Sampson M, Perl S, Young NS, et al. Rosuvastatin alters the proteome of high density lipoproteins: Generation of alpha-1-antitrypsin enriched particles with anti-inflammatory properties. Molecular and Cellular Proteomics. 2015;**14**(12):3247-3257

[38] Javeed R, Jabeen F, Saeed H, Najam-ul-Haq M. Advance workflow in lipoproteomics via polymeric ion exchanger. Analytical Chemistry. 2015; **87**(6):3505-3512

[39] Ljunggren SA, Helmfrid I, Norinder U, Fredriksson M, Wingren G, Karlsson H, et al. Alterations in high-density lipoprotein proteome and function associated with persistent organic pollutants. Environment International. 2017;**98**:204-211

[40] Mendoza S, Trenchevska O, King SM, Nelson RW, Nedelkov D, Krauss RM, et al. Changes in low-density lipoprotein size phenotypes associate with changes in apolipoprotein C-III glycoforms after dietary interventions. Journal of Clinical Lipidology. 2017;**11**(1):224-233

[41] Yang ZH, Gordon SM, Sviridov D, Wang S, Danner RL, Pryor M, et al. Dietary supplementation with long-chain monounsaturated fatty acid isomers decreases atherosclerosis and alters lipoprotein proteomes in LDLr−/− mice. Atherosclerosis. 2017;**262**:31-38

[42] Eroglu A, Schulze KJ, Yager J, Cole RN, Christian P, Nonyane BA, et al. Plasma proteins associated with circulating carotenoids in Nepalese school-aged children. Archives of Biochemistry and Biophysics. 2018;**646**: 153-160

[43] Jain RB, Ducatman A. Associations between lipid/lipoprotein levels and perfluoroalkyl substances among US children aged 6–11 years. Environmental Pollution. 2018;**243** (Pt A):1-8

[44] Ledda C, Iavicoli I, Bracci M, Avola R, Senia P, Santarelli L, et al. Serum lipid, lipoprotein and apolipoprotein profiles in workers exposed to low arsenic levels: Lipid profiles and occupational arsenic exposure. Toxicology Letters. 2018;**282**: 49-56

[45] Gardner MS, Kuklenyik Z, Lehtikoski A, Carter KA, McWilliams LG, Kusovschi J, et al. Development and application of a high

throughput one-pot extraction protocol for quantitative LC-MS/MS analysis of phospholipids in serum and lipoprotein fractions in normolipidemic and dyslipidemic subjects. Journal of Chromatography B. 2019;**1118**:137-147

[46] Ikuta A, Sakurai T, Nishimukai M, Takahashi Y, Nagasaka A, Hui SP, et al. Composition of plasmalogens in serum lipoproteins from patients with non-alcoholic steatohepatitis and their susceptibility to oxidation. Clinica Chimica Acta. 2019;**493**:1-7

[47] Jayaraman S, Baveghems C, Chavez OR, Rivas-Urbina A, Sánchez-Quesada JL, Gursky O. Effects of triacylglycerol on the structural remodeling of human plasma very low- and low-density lipoproteins. Biochimica et Biophysica Acta (BBA)—Molecular and Cell Biology of Lipids. 2019;**1864**(7):1061-1071

[48] Ma L, Chan DC, Ooi EM, Barrett PHR, Watts GF. Fractional turnover of apolipoprotein (a) and apolipoprotein B-100 within plasma lipoprotein (a) particles in statin-treated patients with elevated and normal Lp (a) concentration. Metabolism. 2019;**96**: 8-11

[49] Schilcher I, Ledinski G, Radulović S, Hallström S, Eichmann T, Madl T, et al. Endothelial lipase increases antioxidative capacity of high-density lipoprotein. Biochimica et Biophysica Acta (BBA)—Molecular and Cell Biology of Lipids. 2019;**1864**(10): 1363-1374

[50] Sukhorukov V, Gudelj I, Pučić-Baković M, Zakiev E, Orekhov A, Kontush A, et al. Glycosylation of human plasma lipoproteins reveals a high level of diversity, which directly impacts their functional properties. Biochimica et Biophysica Acta (BBA)—Molecular and Cell Biology of Lipids. 2019;**1864**(5):643-653

[51] Averill M, Rubinow KB, Cain K, Wimberger J, Babenko I, Becker JO, et al. Postprandial remodeling of high-density lipoprotein following high saturated fat and high carbohydrate meals. Journal of Clinical Lipidology. 2020;**14**(1):66-76

[52] Wang S, Wang S, Yu X, Zeng J, Li H, Yang R, et al. Magnetic nanoparticles functionalized with immobilized apolipoprotein antibodies for direct detection of non-high density lipoprotein cholesterol in human serum. Chemical Engineering Journal. 2020; **385**:123465

[53] Chang CT, Yang CY, Tsai FJ, Lin SY, Chen CJ. Mass spectrometry-based proteomic study makes high-density lipoprotein a biomarker for atherosclerotic vascular disease. BioMed Research International. 2015;**2015**: 164846. DOI: 10.1155/2015/164846

[54] Rodriguez-Garcia E, Ruiz-Nava J, Santamaria-Fernandez S, Fernandez-Garcia JC, Vargas-Candela A, Yahyaoui R, et al. Implications of the Mediterranean diet and physical exercise on the lipid profile of metabolically healthy obese women as measured by nuclear magnetic resonance spectroscopy (1H NMR). Chemistry and Physics of Lipids. 2018; **213**:68-75

[55] Starich MR, Tang J, Remaley AT, Tjandra N. Squeezing lipids: NMR characterization of lipoprotein particles under pressure. Chemistry and Physics of Lipids. 2020;**228**:104874. DOI: 10.1016/j.chemphyslip.2020.104874

[56] van Tienhoven-Wind L, Dullaart RP. Low normal thyroid function as a determinant of increased large very low density lipoprotein particles. Clinical Biochemistry. 2015;**48** (7–8):489-494

[57] Gruppen EG, Connelly MA, Dullaart RP. Higher circulating GlycA, a

pro-inflammatory glycoprotein biomarker, relates to lipoprotein-associated phospholipase A2 mass in nondiabetic subjects but not in diabetic or metabolic syndrome subjects. Journal of Clinical Lipidology. 2016;**10**(3): 512-518

[58] Buitenwerf E, Dullaart RP, Kobold ACM, Links TP, Sluiter WJ, Connelly MA, et al. Cholesterol delivery to the adrenal glands estimated by adrenal venous sampling: An in vivo model to determine the contribution of circulating lipoproteins to steroidogenesis in humans. Journal of Clinical Lipidology. 2017;**11**(3):733-738

[59] Needham LL, Smy L, Lee MA, Kunzler TM, Genzen JR. Phlebotomy tube interference with nuclear magnetic resonance (NMR) lipoprotein subclass analysis. Clinica Chimica Acta. 2019; **488**:235-241

[60] Hunter WG, McGarrah RW, Kelly JP, Khouri MG, Craig DM, Haynes C, et al. High-density lipoprotein particle subfractions in heart failure with preserved or reduced ejection fraction. Journal of the American College of Cardiology. 2019; **73**(2):177-186

[61] Pallazola VA, Sathiyakumar V, Ogunmoroti O, Fashanu O, Jones SR, Santos RD, et al. Impact of improved low-density lipoprotein cholesterol assessment on guideline classification in the modern treatment era—Results from a racially diverse Brazilian cross-sectional study. Journal of Clinical Lipidology. 2019;**13**(5):804-811

[62] Salahuddin T, Kittelson J, Tardif JC, Shah PK, Olsson AG, Nicholls SJ, et al. Association of high-density lipoprotein particle concentration with cardiovascular risk following acute coronary syndrome: A case-cohort analysis of the dal-outcomes trial. American Heart Journal. 2020;**221**: 60-66

[63] Tucker B, McClelland RL, Allison MA, Budoff MJ, Wu BJ, Barter PJ, et al. Relationship of fibroblast growth factor 21 levels with inflammation, lipoproteins and non-alcoholic fatty liver disease. Atherosclerosis. 2010;**299**:38-44

[64] Coffin S, Limm M, Cowburn D. Correlation of 13C and 1H chemical shifts in bovine high-density lipoprotein from two-dimensional NMR. Journal of Magnetic Resonance (1969). 1984;**59**(2): 268-274

[65] Morgan PE, Sturgess AD, Hennessy A, Davies MJ. Serum protein oxidation and apolipoprotein CIII levels in people with systemic lupus erythematosus with and without nephritis. Free Radical Research. 2007; **41**(12):1301-1312

[66] Lv P, Zhao M, Liu Y, Jin H, Cui W, Fan C, et al. Apolipoprotein C-III in the high-density lipoprotein proteome of cerebral lacunar infarction patients impairs its anti-inflammatory function. International Journal of Molecular Medicine. 2018;**41**(1):61-68

[67] Vaisar T, Mayer P, Nilsson E, Zhao XQ, Knopp R, Prazen BJ. HDL in humans with cardiovascular disease exhibits a proteomic signature. Clinica Chimica Acta. 2010;**411** (13–14):972-979

[68] Jensen MK, Aroner SA, Mukamal KJ, Furtado JD, Post WS, Tsai MY, et al. HDL subspecies defined by presence of apolipoprotein C-III and incident coronary heart disease in four cohorts. Circulation. 2018;**137**(13):1364

[69] Mangé A, Goux A, Badiou S, Patrier L, Canaud B. HDL proteome in hemodialysis patients: A quantitative nanoflow liquid chromatography-tandem mass spectrometry approach. PLoS One. 2012;**7**(3):e34107. DOI: 10.1371/journal.pone.0034107

[70] Pechlaner R, Tsimikas S, Yin X, Willeit P, Baig F, Santer P, et al. Very-low-density lipoprotein-associated apolipoproteins predict cardiovascular events and are lowered by inhibition of APOC-III. Journal of the American College of Cardiology. 2017;**69**(7): 789-800

[71] Tan Y, Liu TR, Hu SW, Tian D, Li C, Zhong JK, et al. Acute coronary syndrome remodels the protein cargo and functions of high-density lipoprotein subfractions. PLoS One. 2014;**9**(4):e94264. DOI: 10.1371/journal.pone.0094264

[72] Yan LR, Wang DX, Liu H, Zhang XX, Zhao H, Hua L, et al. A pro-atherogenic HDL profile in coronary heart disease patients: An iTRAQ labelling-based proteomic approach. PLoS One. 2014;**9**(5):e98368. DOI: 10.1371/journal.pone.0098368

[73] Natarajan P, Collier TS, Jin Z, Lyass A, Li Y, Ibrahim NE, et al. Association of an HDL apolipoproteomic score with coronary atherosclerosis and cardiovascular death. Journal of the American College of Cardiology. 2019;**73**(17):2135-2145

[74] Marsillach J, Becker JO, Vaisar T, Hahn BH, Brunzell JD, Furlong CE, et al. Paraoxonase-3 is depleted from the high-density lipoproteins of autoimmune disease patients with subclinical atherosclerosis. Journal of Proteome Research. 2015;**14**(5): 2046-2054

[75] Emmens JE, Jones DJ, Cao TH, Chan DC, Romaine SP, Quinn PA, et al. Proteomic diversity of high-density lipoprotein explains its association with clinical outcome in patients with heart failure. European Journal of Heart Failure. 2018;**20**(2):260-267

[76] Gordon SM, Davidson WS, Urbina EM, Dolan LM, Heink A, Zang H, et al. The effects of type 2 diabetes on lipoprotein composition and arterial stiffness in male youth. Diabetes. 2013;**62**(8):2958-2967

[77] Kheniser KG, Osme A, Kim C, Ilchenko S, Kasumov T, Kashyap SR. Temporal dynamics of high-density lipoprotein proteome in diet-controlled subjects with type 2 diabetes. Biomolecules. 2020;**10**(4):520

[78] Manjunatha S, Distelmaier K, Dasari S, Carter RE, Kudva YC, Nair KS. Functional and proteomic alterations of plasma high density lipoproteins in type 1 diabetes mellitus. Metabolism. 2016; **65**(9):1421-1431

[79] Gourgari E, Ma J, Playford MP, Mehta NN, Goldman R, Remaley AT, et al. Proteomic alterations of HDL in youth with type 1 diabetes and their associations with glycemic control: A case-control study. Cardiovascular Diabetology. 2019;**18**(1):43

[80] Holzer M, Wolf P, Curcic S, Birner-Gruenberger R, Weger W, Inzinger M, et al. Psoriasis alters HDL composition and cholesterol efflux capacity. Journal of Lipid Research. 2012;**53**(8): 1618-1624

[81] Watanabe J, Charles-Schoeman C, Miao Y, Elashoff D, Lee YY, Katselis G, et al. Proteomic profiling following immunoaffinity capture of HDL: Association of acute phase proteins and complement factors with pro-inflammatory HDL in rheumatoid arthritis. Arthritis and Rheumatism;**64** (6):1828

[82] Rao PK, Merath K, Drigalenko E, Jadhav AY, Komorowski RA, Goldblatt MI, et al. Proteomic characterization of high-density lipoprotein particles in patients with non-alcoholic fatty liver disease. Clinical Proteomics. 2018;**15**:10. DOI: 10.1186/s12014-018-9186-0

[83] Kim SS, Kim MH, Shin BK, Na HJ, Choi JY, Kee MK, et al. Different

isoforms of apolipoprotein AI present heterologous post-translational expression in HIV infected patients. Journal of Proteome Research. 2007; **6**(1):180-184

[84] Gu JG, Zhu CL, Cheng DZ, Xie Y, Liu F, Zhou X. Enchanced levels of apolipoprotein M during HBV infection feedback suppresses HBV replication. Lipids in Health and Disease. 2011;**10**:154. DOI: 10.1186/1476-511X-10-154

[85] Shen B, Yi X, Sun Y, Bi X, Du J, Zhang C, et al. Proteomic and metabolomic characterization of COVID-19 patient Sera. Cell. 2020; **182**(1):59-72.e15. DOI: 10.1016/j.cell.2020.05.032

[86] Dashty M, Motazacker MM, Levels J, de Vries M, Mahmoudi M, Peppelenbosch MP, et al. Proteome of human plasma very low-density lipoprotein and low-density lipoprotein exhibits a link with coagulation and lipid metabolism. Thrombosis and Haemostasis. 2014;**111**(3):518-530

[87] Davidsson P, Hulthe J, Fagerberg B, Olsson BM, Hallberg C, Dahllof B, et al. A proteomic study of the apolipoproteins in LDL subclasses in patients with the metabolic syndrome and type 2 diabetes. Journal of Lipid Research. 2005;**46**(9):1999-2006

[88] Li D, Huang F, Zhao Y, Villata PW, Griffin TJ, Zhang L, et al. Plasma lipoproteome in Alzheimer's disease: A proof-of-concept study. Clinical Proteomics. 2018;**15**(1):31. DOI: 10.1186/s12014-018-9207-z

[89] Yeung PK. Metabolomics and biomarkers for drug discovery. Metabolites. 2018;**8**(1):11. DOI: 10.3390/metabo8010011

[90] Green PS, Vaisar T, Pennathur S, Kulstad JJ, Moore AB, Marcovina S, et al. Combined statin and niacin therapy remodels the high-density lipoprotein proteome. Circulation. 2008;**118**(12):1259-1267

[91] Okada T, Ohama T, Takafuji K, Kanno K, Matsuda H, Sairyo M, et al. Shotgun proteomic analysis reveals proteome alterations in HDL of patients with cholesteryl ester transfer protein deficiency. Journal of Clinical Lipidology. 2019;**13**(2):317-325

[92] Nagao M, Nakajima H, Toh R, Hirata KI, Ishida T. Cardioprotective effects of high-density lipoprotein beyond its anti-atherogenic action. Journal of Atherosclerosis and Thrombosis. 2018;**25**(10):985-993

[93] Amiri-Dashatan N, Koushki M, Abbaszadeh HA, Rostami-Nejad M, Rezaei-Tavirani M. Proteomics applications in health: Biomarker and drug discovery and food industry. Iranian Journal of Pharmaceutical Research. 2018;**17**(4):1523-1536

Chapter 4

Microarrays and NGS for Drug Discovery

Laura-Ancuta Pop, Oana Zanoaga, Paul Chiroi, Andreea Nutu, Schuyler S. Korban, Cristina Stefan, Alexandru Irimie and Ioana Berindan-Neagoe

Abstract

Novel technologies and state of the art platforms developed and launched over the last two decades such as microarrays, next-generation sequencing, and droplet PCR have provided the medical field many opportunities to generate and analyze big data from the human genome, particularly of genomes altered by different diseases like cancer, cardiovascular, diabetes and obesity. This knowledge further serves for either new drug discovery or drug repositioning. Designing drugs for specific mutations and genotypes will dramatically modify a patient's response to treatment. Among other altered mechanisms, drug resistance is of concern, particularly when there is no response to cancer therapy. Once these new platforms for omics data are in place, available information will be used to pursue precision medicine and to establish new therapeutic guidelines. Target identification for new drugs is necessary, and it is of great benefit for critical cases where no alternatives are available. While mutational status is of highest importance as some mutations can be pathogenic, screening of known compounds in different preclinical models offer new and quick strategies to find alternative frameworks for treating more diseases with limited therapeutic options.

Keywords: NGS, microarray, transcriptomics, drug discovery

1. Introduction

Over the last few decades, major breakthroughs in scientific and technology-related fields have been made, contributing to major gains and significant advances in clinical practices in dealing with cancer diagnosis, treatment, and preventive measures. Although we are now better informed, skilled, and equipped than ever before, efforts for administering effective cancer treatments, and drugs do not appear to have advanced far enough. In spite of all the changes implemented in translational oncology due to availability of new and sophisticated molecular tools, there is a missing link between pre-clinical data and actual findings. Although significant funds have been allocated for pre-clinical studies, 95% of therapeutic strategies have not passed phase I clinical trials in humans. It is likely that those settings prior to drug development may not be adequate enough to effectively mimic human responses. Those few drugs that are approved by regulatory agencies have had either very little or no effects on overall survival rates. Therefore, the lack of efficacy associated with the current anticancer drugs along with the high treatment costs are both contributing to growing incidence and mortality of cancer patients worldwide [1–3].

Cancer, the umbrella term used for a series of more than 200 different neoplastic diseases caused by abnormal cellular divisions due to either singular or cumulative genomic events is, without a doubt, the most dreaded health problem over the past centuries, including current times [4]. According to GLOBOCAN, cancer is one of the leading causes of death, accounting for more than 18 million cases worldwide. These cases are expected to increase by approximately 70% over the next two decades [5–7]. As the incidence of cancer continues to grow, and the disease becomes more difficult to treat, the challenge of discovering new and more effective anticancer drugs is more critical than ever before [8].

From a historical point of view, secondary metabolites extracted from different natural products were the very first known sources of new therapeutic compounds. Early on, the screening process of every novel drug was rather simple, usually based on various ethnobotanical claims, and often fueled by serendipity [9, 10]. However, this traditional approach was soon replaced with modern methods.

With the advent of modern omics technologies, and ever-expanding knowledge of the human genome, as well as of genomes of various organisms, including pathogenic ones, drug discovery has evolved into a therapeutic target-based approach. Moreover, recent computational advances in handling and analysis of big data, particularly of complex biological information, have become more user-friendly and less time-consuming. All these developments have accelerated the process, and have paved the way for the beginning of the modern drug discovery era [9, 11].

Early pioneering discoveries of Claude Bernard, Louis Pasteur, and Robert Koch, followed by significant findings in other disciplines, such as in organic chemistry, have set many milestones by the end of the nineteenth century. These developments have laid the foundations for what it is know as the era of modern drug discovery, one of the most provocative scientific fields. Since then, myriad treatments have become available, and many diseases, including those of viral, bacterial, and parasitic infections, as well as of diabetes and cardiovascular disorders, along with various types of cancer have become either treatable, curable, or at least can be held off at symptomatic levels. Furthermore, modern drug discovery has aided in the identification of several pharmacological compounds that would promote safety of many surgical procedures, and have contributed to successful cell- and solid- organ transplantation [9, 12].

Drug discovery is a very long, challenging, and complex multistep process that can be generally split into four main steps, as follows: target selection and validation; compound screening and lead candidate optimization; preclinical studies; and clinical trials [11]. Although it is highly desirable to develop a rapid and effective treatment for every disease, drug development remains a lengthy process, requiring up to 15 years of work along with millions to billions of dollars simply to turn a single drug candidate into an efficient, safe, and accessible product. In particular, costs for cancer care in the United States are projected to reach up to $246 billion by 2030 (a 34% increase from 2015), while anticancer drug development remains at a high rate of failure [13–15].

Over the past 25 years, benefits of implementing many innovative scientific technologies have been made possible due to advances in molecular research studies prior to anticancer drug discovery [16]. Further, our understanding of cancer biology has significantly expanded, as new molecular strategies have exceeded the expectations, and helped rising the overall patient survival rates [17, 18]. Furthermore, as academic research centers have begun to openly embrace collaborations with pharmaceutical and biotechnology companies, the ecosystem for drug discovery has become more responsive and efficient than ever before. As a result, there have been vast expansions of the chemical compound libraries, well beyond those known natural products that have been exploited in the past. Modern technologies, such as high-throughput screening (HTS), fragment-based screening (FBS), molecular modeling, crystallography, nanotechnology, and advanced chemistry, among others, are also currently playing important roles in the revolution of drug discovery [9, 19].

Next generation sequencing (NGS), also known as massively parallel sequencing, refers to a number of molecular high-throughput methods that follow the same principle of simultaneously deciphering millions of nucleotide sequences in a fast, accurate, and affordable approach. Unlike previous sequencing technologies, a whole genome can be sequenced at once, producing 100-folds more data than other tools based on Sanger's sequencing method. Thus, NGS has become one of the major omics technologies to be adopted in life sciences fields, including functional genomics, metagenomics, transcriptomics, and oncogenomics. Therefore, HTS methods, such as those of the NGS repertory, are expected to notably accelerate drug discovery and reduce associated costs [20, 21].

Another omics technology of interest is that of microarrays, as this tool allows for simultaneous analysis of DNA and assessing of mRNA expression levels. As a result, microarrays have been rapidly exploited in various research studies, including those focused on drug discovery, as they afford a better understanding of both the pathological mechanism and drug activity. Furthermore, microarray technologies are useful in identifying a drug target or a biological compound(s) that may interact with a synthetically designed drug. In addition, the microarray technology is highly efficient and of low-cost, but has some limitations, particularly pertaining to availability of advanced bioinformatic analysis tools [22]. These two omics technologies will be further discussed below.

Overall, the above-mentioned technologies and tools will have major impacts on revolutionizing drug discovery efforts, including identifying more efficacious and effective anticancer drugs in shorter periods of time, and at reduced costs [23].

2. Microarrays and drug discovery

2.1 Microarray technology: role, types, and applications

The microarray technology is powerful though early on it has had some limitations due to its high costs. However, in recent years, it has become more affordable with the availability of commercial microarray chips and platforms. Thus, this technology has moved from research laboratories to clinical applications. In recent years, microarrays have played significant roles in drug discovery. A large number of studies have demonstrated that microarray datasets not only allow for rapid and direct analysis of large amounts of biological information, but these also promote identification of potential biomarkers for various diseases [24–28]. Furthermore, microarray datasets can potentially determine the appropriate drug dose that can maximize its therapeutic effect. In clinical trials, microarrays can be used for early detection of any toxicity or any side-effects of a drug or a drug dose in order to provide rapid, sensitive, and safe treatments. Moreover, microarrays play important roles in pharmacogenomics by allowing for identification of associations between responses to drug treatment and a patient's genetic profile [28, 29], as well as for selecting the most appropriate new candidate drugs for clinical trials.

There are several types of microarrays, including DNA microarrays, microRNA arrays, chemical compound microarrays, antibody microarrays, protein microarrays, tissue microarrays, and carbohydrate arrays. In clinical research, DNA microarrays are often used for novel biomarker discovery [30]. Among other applications of DNA/RNA microarrays are the following: 1) identification of differential gene expression, 2) analysis of mutations, 3) screening of single nucleotide polymorphisms (SNPs), 4) determination of methylation, acetylation, and alternative splicing, and 5) comparative genomic hybridization [31–34].

Microarrays consist of hundreds to thousands of DNA, RNA, oligonucleotides, or other probe molecules that are immobilized in an array format onto a solid support surface, such as microscope glass slides, silicon chips, or nylon membranes, and then exposed to labeled samples carrying corresponding target molecules to allow for simultaneous detection of nucleic acid/protein/antibody/other targets. Typically, a single probe is at one-time leading to a microarray with hundreds of thousands of different oligonucleotide sequences complementary to distinct fragments of known DNA or RNA sequences [35]. Components of a DNA or an RNA sample loaded onto a slide/chip/membrane will hybridize specifically to their complementary probes, and the fluorescence intensity will correspond to the amount of DNA or RNA of a given gene in a sample [36].

Microarrays are processed in either "one-color" or "two-color" formats. In a one-color format, a single RNA sample is labeled with a fluorophore, such as cyanine-3 (Cy-3) or cyanine-5 (Cy-5) prior to hybridization, and the intensity of the fluorophore is determined [37]. Whereas a two-color microarray capitalizes on a competitive hybridization (**Figure 1**). In this format, a single nucleic acid sample is labeled with a green dye, while a related sample is labeled with a red dye. Following hybridization and removal of unbound nucleic acids, a laser scanner will detect those red- and green-labeled molecules. The intensity of each colored spot on an array is determined, and the red/green ratio is determined [38].

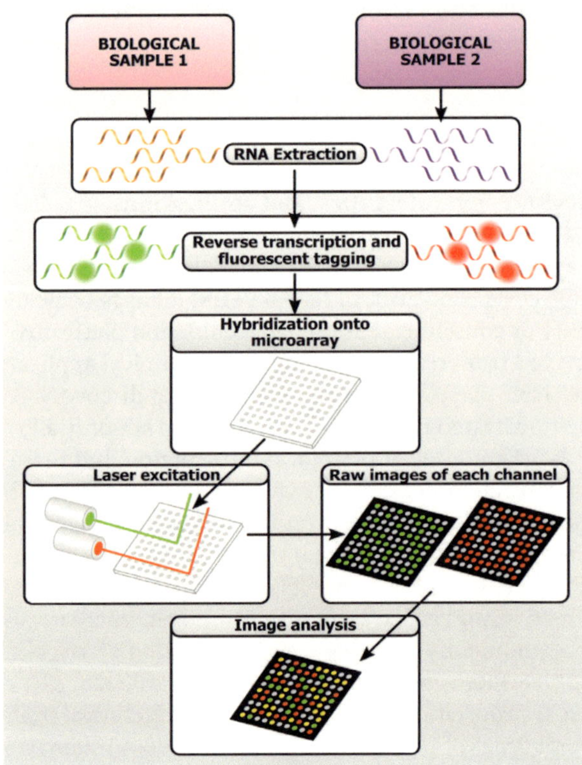

Figure 1.
A general workflow for a typical two-color microarray experiment.

Several microarray technologies have been developed using various platforms that have been optimized to maximize reproducibility and accuracy of findings [39]. For example, Affymetrix GeneChip microarrays are manufactured using photolithography that utilize oligonucleotide probes. This system has the capability of monitoring expression of every gene in a genome. In fact, Affymetrix GeneChips have been used for genotyping, copy number analysis, transcriptome analysis, and miRNA profiling. On the other hand, Agilent oligonucleotide microarrays are based on inkjet technology for *in situ* manufacturing of probes, wherein actual probe sequences are used as linkers in order to extend these probes to provide higher specificity [39]. Whereas, Illumina BeadArrays are based on patterned substrates for high-density detection of target nucleic acids using silica microbeads [40].

Some of the common available techniques used in drug development efforts, including microarrays, are listed in **Table 1**.

2.2 Droplet Digital PCR (ddPCR) and microarrays

The Droplet Digital PCR (ddPCR) is a recent technology that is commercially available, capitalizing on the use of *Taq* polymerase in a standard PCR reaction in order to amplify a target DNA fragment from a complex sample using pre-validated primers or primer/probe assays [61, 62]. Galbiati et al. have proposed a workflow that combined a microarray assay with ddPCR for both detection and quantification of circulating tumor DNA mutations in colon cancer patients [63]. This approach is useful for the development of reliable non-invasive biomarkers for RAS and BRAF mutations, identifying a target mutation, and providing clinically relevant information. Microarray analysis and ddPCR data have identified mutations in primary breast tumors from female patients treated with adjuvant mono-tamoxifen therapy [64]. Moreover, using microarray and ddPCR, it is observed that epidermal growth factor receptor (EGFR) expression can be used as a prognostic biomarker in patients with oropharyngeal squamous cell carcinoma, as it is associated with smoking status [65]. In another study, microarray analysis of uterine tissue, along with validation using ddPCR has allowed for observing downregulation of genes in pathways of

Techniques	Applications	References
ChIP microarrays	Drug development Pharmacogenomics Gene discovery Gene expression profiling	[41–46]
Splice variants	Pharmacogenomics Drug discovery Biomarker identification Polymorphism/SNP detection Drug target identification	[47–52]
Genotyping	Drug discovery Pharmacogenomics Environmental monitoring Drug resistance Vaccine candidate identification	[53–57]
Comparative genomic hybridization (CGH)	Gene discovery Biomarker identification Clinical application Vaccine candidate identification	[29, 52, 58–60]

Table 1.
Available techniques for drug discovery.

the immune response following tetrabromobisphenol A treatment [66]. Moreover, ddPCR analysis of miRNAs identified using a microarray assay has revealed that anti-apoptotic miRNA may be potentially involved in antagonistic effects between the *Alternaria* mycotoxins alternariol and altertoxin *II* in HepG2 cells [67]. In another study using this combined approach, transglutaminase 2 is identified as a novel regulator of the tumor microenvironment in gastric cancer patients, thus serving as a promising target for restricting tumor-promoting inflammation [68].

2.3 Undruggable to druggable proteins using microarrays

In recent years, efforts have been directed towards transforming those proteins that are deemed pharmacologically incapable of being targeted, coined as "undruggable", into "druggable" proteins. Despite the fact that many proteins, such as kinases, that promote cancer development, are capable of serving as drug targets, proteins such as RAS, MYC, and p53 are deemed as "undruggable targets" [69]. Thus, overcoming these "undruggable targets" becomes one of the main challenges for drug discovery. One of the new proposed methods to overcome these challenges is represented by the inhibition of kinase activities of oncogenic proteins using small molecules and antibodies [70]. In one approach, blocking of pathways downstream of a target protein has served as a viable strategy to assess the functional role of a mutation as an oncogenic driver of different types of cancers, and for serving as a valid clinical trial design [71]. In another approach, discovery of hidden allosteric sites is an effective strategy for development of new drug targets, as well as for discovery of allosteric drugs [69].

It is known that *RAS* mutations serve as early genetic events in tumor progression, while sustained expression of *RAS* mutations are deemed necessary for tumor maintenance [72]. Although RAS have been deemed as "undruggable", recent studies have demonstrated that therapies targeting either RAS-activating pathways or RAS effectors pathways combined with direct RAS inhibitors, along with immune checkpoint inhibitors or T-cell targeting methods, *RAS*-mutant tumors are found to be treatable [73]. As the transcription factor MYC promotes cancer progression, small-molecule inhibitors are used to drug the "undruggable" by inducing epigenetic silencing and regulating G-quadruplex structures within the *MYC* promoter [74]. In another example, *p53* is well known as the most frequently altered gene in human cancer, and therefore the p53 mutant protein is deemed as an important undruggable target [75]. Such compounds as p53 reactivation, induction of massive apoptosis-1 (PRIMA-1), and a structural analogue of PRIMA-1, APR-246, have been found to reactivate the mutant p53 protein by converting it to a form with wild-type properties [75].

Using a custom-designed lncRNA microarray, Orilnc1 was identified as a novel nonprotein mediator of RAS/RAF activation, with potential applications as a therapeutic target in RAS/RAF-driven cancers [76]. An Affymetrix microarray revealed coexpression of a mutant β-catenin and K-Ras in mice by targeting β-catenin in hepatocellular cancers [77]. Microarray and pathway enrichment analyses revealed that MYC expression could be downregulated by 1,2,3,4,6-penta-O-galloyl-beta-D-glucopyranoside (PGG) in hepatocellular carcinoma [78]. Using a genome-wide microarray analysis, it was reported that targeting c-Myc would unlock novel strategies to combat asthma [79]. β-catenin could be deemed as an anticancer therapeutic target by regulating c-Myc and CDKN1A expression in breast cancer cells [80]. In addition, microarray data identified and characterized novel p53 target genes expressed in hepatocarcinoma cells, and were associated with steroid hormones processing and transfer [81]. Furthermore, it was proposed that there was a novel non-cell-autonomous tumor-suppressive regulation, mediated by p53, playing a key role in maintaining organism homeostasis. Moreover, breast cancer metastasis suppressor 1-like (BRMS1L) was found to be upregulated by p53 protein. In addition, p53 inhibited cancer cell invasion and migration, and thus could serve as a therapeutic target for cancer [82].

2.4 Microarrays and drug resistance

Resistance to chemotherapy remains a major obstacle to improving a cancer patient's outcome and survival despite significant advances in surgery, radiation therapy, and anticancer treatments. In cancer, drug resistance arises from a complex range of molecular and biochemical processes, such as modifications in DNA repair mechanism, drug uptake, absorption, and metabolism. Recent studies have identified two forms of drug resistance in cancer patients, intrinsic (innate resistance that is present before a patient is exposed to drugs) and acquired (a direct result of chemotherapy). A growing number of microarray studies have exploited the identification of mechanisms involved in both drug response and drug resistance in clinical samples in order to identify biomarkers for drug resistance [83]. For example, microarray analysis has provided a better understanding of circular RNA expression profiles that are associated with gemcitabine resistance in pancreatic cancer cells [84]. In human gastric cancer tissues, a microarray study has revealed that miR-424 regulates cisplatin resistance of gastric cancer [85]. Furthermore, extracellular matrix proteins have been implicated in drug-resistant ovarian cancer cells, thus inhibiting penetration of a drug into cells, as well as contributing to increased apoptosis resistance [86].

Of particular interest, new genes associated with drug resistance development in ovarian cancer have been discovered using microarray analysis, wherein 13 genes are found to be upregulated, while nine genes are found to be downregulated [87]. In triple-negative breast cancer cells, notable alterations are observed at both transcriptomic and genomic levels, along with identification of a mutation (*TP53*) associated with drug response [88]. In another study, bioinformatics analyses of microarray datasets have identified neuromedin U (NMU) as a potential gene that confers alectinib resistance in non-small cell lung cancer [89]. Furthermore, expression profiling has allowed for discovery of genes involved in ovarian-drug resistance, wherein these genes are found to be controlled via different signaling pathways, including MAPK–Akt, Wnt, and Notch [90]. In another study, microarray analysis has found that tumor initiation and insulin-like growth factor (IGF)/fibroblast growth factor (FGF) signaling contribute to sorafenib resistance in hepatocellular carcinoma [91].

As antibiotic resistance has become a global health problem, efforts are underway to identify and screen for new and effective antibiotics. A microarray for 132 gram-negative bacteria has been evaluated to detect genes for resistance to 75 clinically relevant antibiotics [92]. Frye et al. have developed a DNA microarray capable of detecting all antimicrobial resistance genes found at the National Center for Biotechnology [93]. Furthermore, a microarray has been use to identify *Helicobacter pylori* resistance to clarithromycin and levofloxacin, as well as to detect *CYP2C19* polymorphism [94]. It is reported that this microarray can be used for individual therapy detection as it has high specificity, reproducibility, and sensitivity [78]. In another study, an effort has been successfully undertaken to reduce antibiotic susceptibility testing assay time, as well as for rapid determination of minimum inhibitory concentrations of different antibiotics using a nanoliter-sized microchamber/microarray-based microfluidic (N-3 M) platform [95]. More recently, a commercially available microarray (IDENTIBAC AMR-ve) has been developed for determination of antibiotic-resistant clinical isolates of *Klebsiella pneumoniae,* and to identify genes associated with resistance to a wide range of antibiotics [96].

2.5 Identifying new drugs using microarray

Microarrays have been successfully used not only in various fields of medical research and for treatment, but also as useful platforms/tools for drug discovery. A general scheme for drug discovery and development is presented in **Figure 2**.

Small-molecule microarrays (SMMs) serve as a robust and novel technology that will have important applications in target-based drug discovery. In this technology, it is proposed that depending on the screening strategy, small molecules are either covalently or noncovalently immobilized onto a microchip. Hence, high precision robotic printers are used to automatically spot around 5000 molecules along a standard microscopic glass slide, with a spot diameter ranging between 80 and 200 μm. Therefore, a biomolecule of interest is tagged with a fluorophore, and then detected through a fluorescence-based readout. Using this SMM technology on a mammary tumor organoid model, multiple Malat1 ENE triplex-binding chemotypes have been identified, and selected compounds have been found to reduce expression levels of *MALAT1* [97]. This effort has demonstrated the plausibility of designing small molecules to investigate and treat *MALAT1*-driven type cancers.

An AbsorbArray is a small molecule microarray-based approach that allows for unmodified compounds to noncovalently adhere onto surfaces of an agarose-coated microarray to bind to RNA-motif libraries in a massively parallel format [98]. Using this platform, Hafeez et al. have designed a small molecule (TGP-377) that specifically and potently enhances vascular endothelial growth factor a (*VEGFA*) expression by targeting miR-377 and *VEGFA* mRNA [99].

Over the past decade, various drug screening platforms have been developed to control delivery of different drug candidates into target cells, including drug patterning, stamping, and microfluidic loading [100]. For example, a microarray-based screening system to test for effects of small molecules on mammalian cells utilizes an imaging-based readout. This system allows for conducting small-molecule screening for discovery of new chemical tools and of potential therapeutic agents [101]. In another example, a printed hydrogel is used in a high-throughput microarray-based

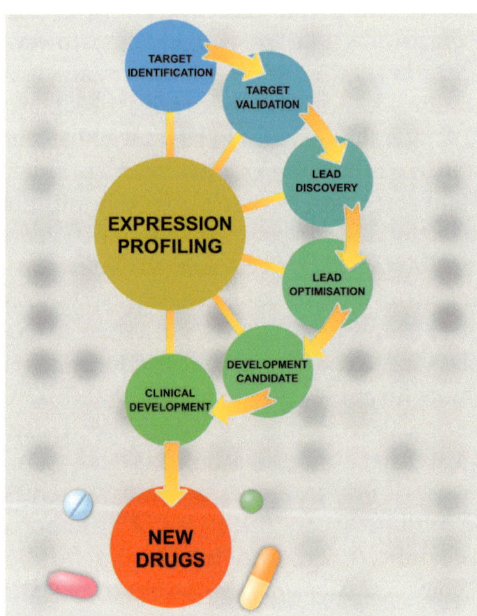

Figure 2.
Major steps undertaken in discovery and development of new drugs.

screening platform for rapidly and inexpensively identification of clinically promising lead compounds with inhibitory potentials [86]. Moreover, this platform can be used to quantify dose–response relationships of such inhibitors [102].

A schematic diagram of the drug discovery process using microarrays is presented in **Figure 2**.

2.6 Microarrays and drug discovery for cancer

Microarrays are playing important roles in the discovery of critical drugs for the treatment of various forms of cancer. An overview of the scheme for anticancer drug discovery and development using microarrays is presented in **Figure 3**.

Microarray-based mRNA expression analysis has revealed that artemisinin induced iron-dependent cell death (ferroptosis) in an NCI cell line panel [103]. In this study, genes subjected to cluster analysis have been derived from different microarray hybridization platforms (Stanford, Affymetrix U95U95v2, U133, and U133A/U133) [87]. It is observed that *OGFOD1* and *TFRC* genes have exhibited comparable responses in Affymetrix microarrays U133 and U133A/U133B. In another microarray analysis study including 293 stomach tumor tissues and 196 normal tissues, it is found that two hub genes, Serpin Family E Member 1 (*SERPINE1*) and Secreted Protein Acidic and Cysteine Rich (*SPARC*), are significantly upregulated in gastric tissues, and are associated with poor outcomes [88]. Thus, this has demonstrated that transcriptome microarray datasets may facilitate early diagnosis of gastric cancer, and they may be used for pursuing effective treatment approaches [104].

Interestingly, scopoletin, a coumarin compound, is found to have an antiproliferative activity against tumor cells with ABC-transporter expression [89]. Furthermore, COMPARE and hierarchical cluster analysis of transcriptome-wide mRNA expression have supported the capacity of such compounds in drug development [105].

Furthermore, microarray analysis has provided evidence that the micro-RNA has-miR-542-5p can serve as a predictive biomarker, as well as a potential target for therapy in breast cancer [106]. Moreover, this microRNA acts via a mechanism involving the following target genes *YWHAB*, *LY9*, and *SFRP1* [90]. In another

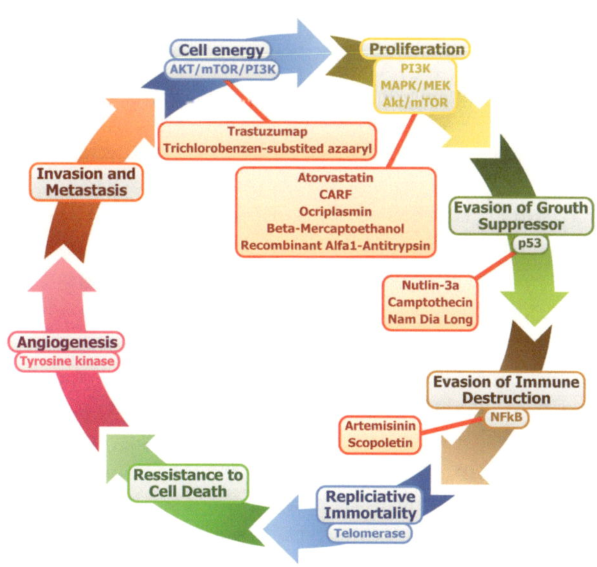

Figure 3.
The hallmarks of cancer and drug discovery using microarrays.

study, it is reported that for patients with high-grade gliomas, microarray data from GSE4412 and GSE7696 datasets have identified differentially expressed prognostic genes between long-term and short-term survivors [91]. Thus, these genes have been deemed as potential biomarkers for prognostic, diagnostic, and therapeutic strategies [107]. Interestingly, atorvastatin treatment of HepG2 cells is reported to modulate 13 miRs identified in a microarray study [108].

Over the years, there have been several advances in design and analysis of microarray. For example, such advances have helped in the development of more specific biomarkers for prostate cancer in order to design effective therapeutic strategies [109]. It is found that urinary prostate cancer-derived exosomes could serve as promising sources of novel biomarker(s). In another study, fabrication of a microarray platform via a sandwich system has allowed for screening of 320 drug candidates as potential anti-cancer agents in *in vitro* experiments performed on MCF-7 breast cancer cells [110]. Furthermore, new bioinformatics tools have been used for microarray data analysis, and have led to the identification of *CDX2* as a prognostic marker for stages II and III colon cancer [111].

Interestingly, lncRNA-TTN-AS1, a novel vital regulator of esophageal squamous cell carcinoma, has been identified using microarray analysis, and found to correlate with overall survival [96]. This biomarker promotes *SNAIL1* and *FSCN1* expression binding to miR-133b, as well as interaction with mRNA, thereby leading to activation of a metastasis cascade [112]. Carstens et al. have developed a combinatorial chemotherapeutic drug-eluting microarray for tumor-initiating cancer stem cells capable of performing chemosensitivity screens using limited cell numbers [113]. In fact, a lncRNA microarray analysis using hepatocarcinoma HCC cells has demonstrated that HNF1A-AS1 is a direct transactivation target of *HNF1α*, and it may have beneficial effects in the treatment of this form of cancer [114]. A pathway analysis of microarray data has identified a transient receptor potential vanilloid (*TRPV*) 2 as a novel therapeutic target for esophageal squamous cell carcinoma. *TRPV2* depletion is found to down-regulate WNT/β-catenin signaling-related genes, as well as basal cell carcinoma signaling-related genes [115]. In another development, using small molecule microarrays, protein–protein interaction inhibitors of *BRCA1* that can be directly administered to tumor cells have been identified [100]. In fact, these compounds have proven to be useful in cancer therapy by targeting BRCA1/PARP-related pathways involved in DNA damage and repair response [116].

In other cancer drug discovery studies, analysis of microarray data has revealed that manzamine (or Manz A) is found to have an antiproliferative effect on human colorectal carcinoma cells, wherein it reduces expression of genes involved in cell survival, induces apoptotic cell death, and inactivates epithelial to mesenchymal transition (EMT) [117]. Furthermore, Manz A is proposed as a potential anticancer drug for colorectal cancer patients by blocking tumors undergoing EMT process and developing distal metastasis. In another effort, the Collaborator of ARF (CARF) protein has been discovered by microarray analysis as a new target of miR-451, and that it mediates its tumor suppressor function both in normal and stressed biological states [118].

In a comparative study, RNA-seq and qPCR-based arrays were found to be better suited than transcriptomic cDNA microarrays in assessing G protein-coupled receptor (*GPCR*) expression with implications for *GPCR* biology and drug discovery [119]. A gene expression omnibus (GEO) database for mRNA microarray data was used for discovery of potential biomarkers in HER-2 positive breast cancer patients who received a neoadjuvant trastuzumab treatment [120]. Furthermore, a combination therapy of trastuzumab and anti-Wnt or hormone therapy could serve as an effective treatment for breast cancer. In addition, expression microarray analysis led to the identification of internalizing antibodies (CD73 mAbs) for basal breast cancer cells [121]. Thus, these mAbs were found to bind to basal-like breast cancer cell surface receptors of high affinity and specificity, as well as promoted receptor-mediated endocytosis with potential applications in basal-like breast cancer treatment [106]. Following microarray gene expression profile analysis, ocriplasmin, β-mercaptoethanol, and recombinant α 1-antitrypsin were identified as potential drugs for the treatment of papillary thyroid cancer [122]. Moreover, microarray profiling assisted in identifying the cytotoxicity mode of action involved in apoptosis of MCF-7 cells following treatment with Nam Dia Long (NDL), a Vietnamese traditional formula [123].

In other studies, genomics and proteomics data have revealed that the ribonucleotide reductase regulatory subunit M2 (*RRM2*) is a novel target of sorafenib in hepatocellular carcinoma [124]. Whereas, a cDNA microarray analysis has identified trichlorobenzene-substituted azaaryl compounds as novel *FGFR* inhibitors with capabilities in downregulating genes associated with cell cycle progression, and in upregulating genes associated with autophagy pathway in bladder cancer [125].

2.7 Microarrays and drug discovery for various other pathologies

Microarrays have been widely used for screening, identifying, and discovery of drugs for various pathologies. A summary of various microarrays used in the discovery of relevant drugs for some of these pathologies will be presented.

A pharmacogenomics corticosteroid model in rat liver was quantified using microarrays and mass spectrometry-based proteomics [126]. Furthermore, corticosteroid-regulated gene expression was observed at mRNA and protein levels, and acting via mechanisms influencing key turnover processes. In another study, an Affymetrix DMET Plus GeneChip microarray platform was found to be useful in discovery of new genetic variants involved in risperidone-induced hyperprolactinemia based on correlations of genetic variations with target genes of interest [127]. In yet another innovative approach, baseline blood sample microarray data and machine learning were exploited to develop a predictive model for lithium treatment response in bipolar patients based on pre-treatment gender and gene expression data [128]. In fact, this predictive model can be extended not only for other therapeutic drug classes, but also for discovery of new biomarkers [113].

Using an Affymetrix_Hugene_1.0_ST microarray, latrophilin (LPHN) receptors have been identified as novel bronchodilator targets for asthma [114]. Moreover, a single nucleotide polymorphism (SNP) in *LPHN1* correlated with asthma along with higher *LPHN1* expression in lung tissue [129]. Just as important, microarrays, based on normalized cDNA libraries, have been used to successfully discover novel genes as potential candidates for drug targeting. In one study whereby a mouse model of immunoglobulin A nephropathy was used, the single most important drug targets in nephritis, namely up-regulated G-protein coupled receptors (*GPCR*s), have been identified [130]. In other efforts, novel biomarkers related to ageing and age-related diseases have been also discovered using microarrays. For example, Lamb et al. generated a large public database of signatures of drugs and of genes by identifying small molecules with potential applications for the treatment of Alzheimer's disease [131]. Likewise, a microarray study was conducted to compare gene expression of major metabolic tissues in mice, rats, and obese cynomolgus monkeys, and it was observed that a modified growth differentiation factor 15 (GDF15)-Fc fusion proteins could serve as potential therapeutic agents for obesity, and for treatment of related comorbidities [132]. Moreover, chemical microarray-assisted high-throughput screening of potential drugs has contributed for rapid identification of four peptoids as fibroblast growth factor receptors (FGFR) agonists with potential applications in clinical use [113].

In a new twist, a phenotypic microarray (PM) technology has been used to measure *Candida albicans* metabolic activity in the presence/absence of acetylcholine, thus paving the way for discovery and screening of compound libraries for novel anti-fungal drugs [133]. While glycan microarrays were found useful in supporting analysis of receptor-binding specificity for glycan-binding pathogens to tackle viral infections, as well as for appropriate design of viral vectors for therapeutic applications [134, 135]. Along the lines of combining different technologies, microarrays were integrated with high-throughput proteomics to promote discovery of transthyretin as a potentially valuable target for rhabdomyolysis-induced acute kidney injury, as transthyretin induced apoptosis by decreasing accumulation of reactive oxygen species (ROS) [136]. In another study, microarray analysis revealed that the nitric oxide–sensitive soluble guanylyl cyclase improved both diastolic cardiac function and hemodynamics, as well as decreased susceptibility to ventricular arrhythmias in animal models [137]. Whereas, Takahiro et al. reported on a novel method to analyze glycan profiles of hemagglutinin using a lectin microarray that served as a highly sensitive and simple tool for glycan profiling of viral glycoproteins [138]. Similarly, using a high-density peptide microarray, designed using linear peptides and consequentially conformational epitopes, specific diagnostic peptides for the Zika virus were identified, and this approach could be rapidly adapted to other pathogens [139]. In another microarray study along with use of the WGCNA (weighted gene co-expression network analysis) method, genes related to inflammatory and immune responses with critical roles in rheumatoid arthritis pathogenesis have been identified, and both sanguinarine and papaverine were deemed as having potential therapeutic effects on rheumatoid arthritis [140].

In another innovative approach, a meta-analysis of polymyositis and dermatomyositis microarray data has revealed that four novel genes and ten SNP-variant regions could be used either as candidates for potential drug targets or as biomarkers [141]. Interestingly, microarray analyses have indicated that SAM-competitive EZH2 inhibitors in cancer cells induced genes related to cholesterol homeostasis in hepacellular carcinoma [142]. Moreover, gene expression microarray studies have that revealed that T2DM-connected genes as alternative drug targets. Furthermore, interatomic and toxicogenomic have helped to identify signaling pathways involved in disease pathophysiology [143]. An integrative gene expression microarray meta-analysis has provided valuable information about novel potential host factors that can modulate chronic HBV infection, and may serve as potential targets for the development of novel therapeutics such as the activin receptor-like kinase inhibitor [144].

In other innovative platforms, non-natural amino acid peptide microarrays were developed for discovery of Ebola virus glycoprotein affinity ligands, and this system could be used for rapid development of peptide-based antivirals for other diseases [145]. On the other hand, Kusi-Appiah et al. developed a method in order to generate quantitative dose–response curves from microarrays of liposomal small molecules [129]. This method was found to control dosages of small lipophilic molecules provided to cells by varying sub-cellular volumes of surface-supported lipid micro- and nano-structure arrays manufactured using nanointaglio printing [146].

In other studies, microarrays have been used to select either cooperative or non-cooperative peptide pairs for modulating enzyme functions for use in both drug discovery and biocatalysis [147]. Specifically, new peptides promoting inhibition of the target enzyme are selected by jointly using them along with a primary inhibitory peptide. Furthermore, a quantitative PCR-based microarray has been used to assess differences in expression levels of miRNA from plasma of women with or without endometriosis, and a potential diagnostic marker, hsa-miRNA-154-5p, for this disease is identified [148]. In another study, altered gene expression profiles in peripheral blood mononuclear cells (PBMCs) of type 1 diabetes (T1D) are identified using integrated analysis of different microarray studies, thereby offering a new strategy for either preserving or improving β-cell function [149]. Moreover, microarray analysis has allowed for the identification of an aurora kinase A (AURKA) gene involved in cell cycle regulation that could serve as a potential biomarker for predicting poor prognosis in liposarcoma [150].

Microarrays have been used to identify drugs for various other diseases. For example, collagenase is demonstrated to play an important role in ischemia stroke through TNF and IL1B, and a DNA microarray has identified anakinra and nitric oxide as small molecule drugs that are closely associated with this disease [151]. While protein microarrays have been used as platforms to "target hop", critical for identifying small molecules that bind to, and compete with, domain–motif interactions [152]. In fact, Bae et al. have used this platform to identify a novel compound, EML405, via its interaction with the Tudor domain-containing protein Spindlin1, SPIN1. Furthermore, microarray screening has identified a retinoid derivative Tp8 that promotes anti-hepatitis C virus activity via restoration of the gastrointestinal glutathione peroxidase (GI-GPx) [153]. In a different study, a small–molecule microarray (SMM)–based screening has contributed to the identification of an inhibitor (a degradation product from a commercial screening collection) of the "undruggable" small ubiquitin–like modifier (SUMO) E2 enzyme Ubc9 [154]. This latter discovery provides a viable example of the significant pharmacological importance of this SMM screening strategy.

There are additional examples of the impact of microarray analyses in identifying valuable drugs against serious human diseases. GSE7621 microarray data from the GEO database have allowed for the identification of 49 novel small molecular drugs that can target several sub-pathways of Parkinson's disease [155]. Moreover, this strategy has allowed for predicting potential therapeutic properties of novel agents, such as ketoconazole and astemizole, in Parkinson's disease via targeting of key enzymes in the arachidonic acid metabolism [138]. In another microarray study, cyclosporine, ethinyl, and tretinoin have been identified, using the Linear Models for Microarray package, as potential targets for treating pulmonary thromboembolism [156]. Whereas, the effect of astragalosides (AST) in rheumatoid arthritis has been elucidated following microarray analysis of critical differentially expressed lncRNAs involved in this disease, wherein four lncRNAs have been selected as critical therapeutic targets for AST [157]. In a recent study, microarray analysis has revealed that the synthetic lipid AM251 inhibits SMAD2/3 and p38 mitogen-activated protein kinase (MAPK), as well as suppresses EMT of renal tubular epithelial cells [158]. Whereas emodin, a Chinese herb-derived compound, is found to suppress excessive responses of macrophages, and it is capable of restoring macrophage homeostasis in different pathologies [159]. Moreover, findings of a microarray analysis have revealed that medroxyprogesterone acetate (MPA), a progestin-based hormonal contraceptive designed to mimic progesterone, increases expression of genes related to inflammation and cholesterol synthesis, as well as those genes associated with both innate immunity and HIV-1 susceptibility [160]. Finally, integrative microarray data have been exploited to identify eight hub genes and one potential nanomedicinal drug, Selenocysteine, that promotes cartilage regeneration [161].

3. Next generation sequencing for drug discovery

Next generation sequencing (NGS) is the term used for massive parallel sequencing experiments that can be conducted using DNA, RNA, or miRNA. NGS has revolutionized clinical and research studies by enabling sequencing of whole human genomes within a single day.

This powerful NGS can be used in several different areas. For example, NGS can be used in clinical settings for identifying genetic variants with high specificity and sensibility, thus allowing for detection of mosaic mutations that could not be previously identified by Sanger sequencing [162]. In the field of microbiology, NGS can be used for identifying and characterizing pathogens, including novel strains or mutants, thereby allowing for linking a pathogen or a new pathogenic strain to an outbreak in a specific region or to a particular individual(s) [163]. The role of NGS in the field of oncology is quite significant, as this technology can be used for pursuing personalized medicine, in particular for developing targeted therapies for specific cancers correlated with individual genetic profiles of patients. Moreover, NGS is highly useful for diagnosis, and for classification of different types of cancer in both adults and children [162, 164, 165].

Furthermore, NGS is highly versatile, primarily for the diversity of analysis that can be undertaken, as well as to numbers and types of biological samples that can be analyzed. A listing of major types of analyses that can be undertaken, as well as of types of biological samples used in NGS are presented in **Table 2**.

As for drug discovery, NGS has been successfully used in various areas of drug discovery, beginning with target identification, compound screening,

Analysis type	Purpose(s)	Biological sample(s)
Targeted gene sequencing	Identify genetic alteration(s) for a specific set of gene region(s) or SNP(s)	Cell cultures; whole blood; serum; plasma; fresh/frozen tissue; formalin-fixed paraffin-embedded tissue
Whole exome sequencing	Evaluate variation(s) present in coding region(s) of DNA (exomes)	Cell cultures; whole blood; fresh/frozen tissue; formalin-fixed paraffin-embedded tissue
Whole genome sequencing	Identify variations present in the whole genome of an organism(s)	Cell cultures; whole blood; fresh/frozen tissue; formalin-fixed paraffin-embedded tissue
miRNAseq	Identify miRNAs and their expression level(s)	Cell cultures; whole blood; serum; plasma; fresh/frozen tissue
RNAseq	Determine expression levels of whole genes present in an organism	Cell cultures, Whole blood, serum, plasma, fresh/frozen tissue
CHIPseq	Chromatin immunoprecipitation sequencing allows for identifying alterations at DNA –binding sites of different transcriptional factor(s) or protein(s)	Cell cultures; fresh/frozen tissue
Copy number alterations/variations (CNVs)	Detect duplication(s), deletion(s), translocation(s), or inversion(s) of one or more genes	Cell cultures; whole blood; fresh/frozen tissue; formalin-fixed paraffin-embedded tissue
Methylation sequencing	Evaluate whole methylation pattern(s) in CpG, CHG, and CHH regions across a genome	Cell cultures; whole blood; fresh/frozen tissue; formalin-fixed paraffin-embedded tissue

Table 2.
Types of NGS analysis, purpose(s), and biological samples used.

biomarker discovery, identification of biopharmaceuticals, drug resistance, and vaccine discovery [166–168]. Those steps involved in drug discovery where NGS could be of particular use are presented in **Figure 4**.

3.1 Target identification

In recent years, NGS has been valuable in the identification of different genetic alterations of a pathogen/pathology that can be useful for targeted treatment. The versatility of NGS allows for evaluating genomic regions using genomic analysis, transcriptomics, RNAseq, and miRNA seq in order to identify gene(s) and their regulation(s)/functionality(ies) in response to different disease conditions, which in turn could be used for target identification [169].

Analysis of genetic variant(s) is yet another important approach for identifying mutations in rare diseases, as these could then be used for treatment of such target(s) [170, 171]. Epigenetic studies, such as methylation analysis or CHIP-seq analysis, known to be altered in different pathologies, could also aid in identifying targets for specialized treatments/therapies [172, 173].

NGS has been widely used for gene to target identification for treatment of cancer. As it is well known, the National Comprehensive Cancer Network (NCCN) has several guidelines for NGS target identification used for treatment of various types of cancer. These include targeting genes for lung cancer (*EGFR, ALK, ROS1, BRAF*, and *PDL1*) [174], colorectal cancer (*NRAS/HRAS/KRAS, BRAF*, *HER2*, *MLH1, MSH2, MSH6,* and *PMS2*) [175], breast and ovarian cancers (*BRCA1/2, TP53, STK11, PTEN, CDH1, PALB2*, among others) [176]. By identifying mutations in each of these genes, clinicians are able to treat patients with specific targeted treatments. In Waldenström's macroglobulinemia, NGS has been employed in evaluating genomic variations that could better inform treatment of patients, and that would ultimately lead to better outcomes. It is observed that patients with recurrent somatic mutations in genes of myeloid differentiation factor 88 (*MYD88*) and chemokine receptor type 4 (*CXCR4*) demonstrate different responses to the same treatment, and thus these genes serve as clinical determinants of clinical

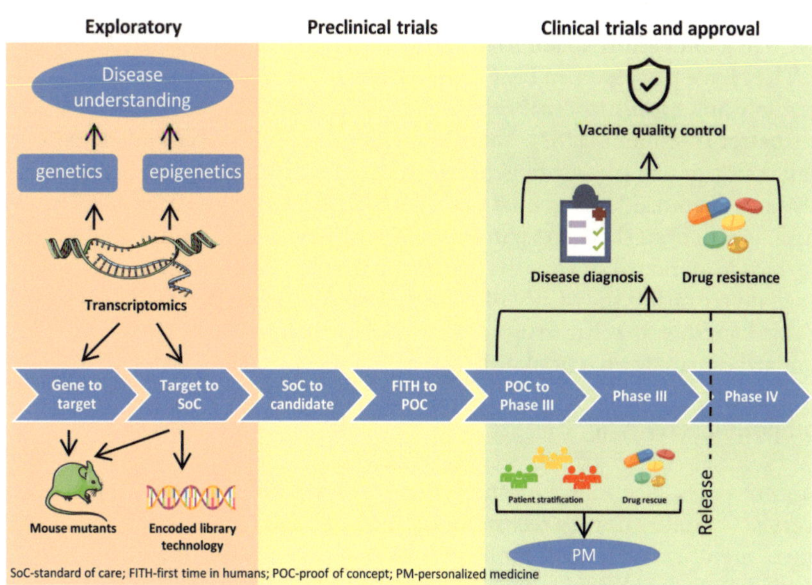

Figure 4.
Various steps involved in drug discovery whereby NGS can be of particular benefit.

presentation [154]. Therefore, a treatment algorithm can be used, based on the mutational status of a patient, in a clinic to adjust targeted treatment [177].

Although cancer has been the most widely studied disease over the last decade, other diseases have employed this approach to identify improved therapies/treatments for each individual patient. For example, Tshibangu-Kabamba et al. have used NGS for evaluating antimicrobial resistance (AMR) of different strains of *Helicobacter pylori*, as well as for determining antimicrobial susceptibilities of these bacterial strains [155]. Whole genome sequencing has aided in identifying several variants in AMR genes, such as *pbp1A* (T558S, F366L), *gyrA* (A92T, A129T), *gyrB* (R579C), and *rdxA* (R131_K166del). This has been instrumental in determining susceptibility of these strains to specific drugs [178].

RNA-seq technology has been used for profiling of host, bacteria, and SARS-CoV-2 virus outbreaks in New York City [156]. It is reported that RNA-seq results are similar to those of RT-PCR. In addition, it is observed that SARS-CoV-2 samples seem to carry other types of viruses. Interestingly, it is also observed that there are gene expression dysregulation in viral response pathways, innate immune responses, and interferon signaling that could explain different responses of patients to the same antiviral drugs [179].

In another study, NGS has been used to identify a targeted treatment for a patient suffering from an immune dysregulation syndrome. As a result, a new germline mutation in the *CTLA4* (Cytotoxic T-Lymphocyte Associated Protein 4) gene, susceptible to the drug abatacept, has been identified [180].

3.2 Target to standard of care

In this step of drug discovery, NGS plays an important role, mainly due to its ability to assess multiple gene alterations within a short period of time. Moreover, the Food and Drug Administration (FDA) has approved NGS testing in clinics. One such example is the case of using a hybrid capture NGS assay for evaluating non-small cell lung cancer in patients. Using this assay, Schatz et al. have diagnosed 417 patients based on both genetic alterations and tumor burden. This approach has made it possible to use specific treatments based on tumor burden values if no actionable genetic alteration is detected [181, 182]. Furthermore, Klowak et al. have used NGS in a pilot study to identify pathogens in neonates suspected of having sepsis. They have proposed an NGS-based protocol for implementation in clinics to accurately and rapidly identify those pathogens affecting neonates, as well as to provide better treatments [183]. Yet in another example, an NGS panel, consisting of seven fusion genes and seven genes with frequent copy number changes, has been used to diagnose 113 sarcoma patients with 97% sensitivity and 100% specificity. This has rendered this gene panel as a highly promising toll for implementing gene targets in standard of care for sarcoma patients [184]. There are several other studies demonstrating the utility of NGS testing in identifying targets that could be actionable by either specific drugs or that could be implemented as specific targets for standard of care for particular diseases [185–189].

3.3 Compound screening

In recent years, a common method used for compound screening during drug discovery is "encoded library technology" (ELT) [190]. ELT is based on DNA binding to members of a small molecule library of chemical compounds. This DNA tag, serving as an amplifiable identification barcode, is unique to each compound/organic ligand, thus rendering it possible for its incubation with specific protein targets of interest. Subsequently, these organic compounds/ligands are washed away based on their affinities to the target; thus, compounds/ligands with high affinities for the target are enriched, and identified by NGS sequencing of PCR products [190]. This approach allows for both constructing and screening of combinatorial libraries of large volumes, thus facilitating rapid discovery of ligands to various different protein targets. ELT is used in several clinical areas, mainly for cancer, but also for various diseases, as it is a rapid and economical screening system of organic compounds [191–194].

Recently, Lemke et al. used ELT and virtual computation library screening methods, DNA-encoded chemical libraries (DECL), to identify inhibitors for poly-ADR-ribose polymerase member 10 (*PARP10*). In effect, they integrated DECL screening with structure-based computational methods to streamline the development of leading compounds. Thus, following DECL screening, they observed that a compound with an A82-CONHMe-B54 motif yielded the best result. Therefore, they screened over 10,500 virtual compounds, and selected ten compounds for synthesis. These compounds were assessed for *PARP10* inhibition, and they found two compounds with promising results [195]. In another study, Reidenbach et al. attempted to identify compounds against Prion disease, a neurodegenerative disease with no therapeutic options; however, the only benzimidazole compounds identified demonstrated low affinities [196]. Whereas, Cuozzo et al. screened a DECL library of 225 million compounds, and identified a single compound (X-165) with a high activity against the production of lysophosphatidic acid, and this compound has been approved by the FDA for Phase I Clinical trials [197]. In other examples of using this strategy, Dawadi et al. discovered a thrombin inhibitor using DECL [198], while, Kung et al. identified two compounds that presented inhibition/binders to e Nα-terminal acetyltransferase (Naa50) using ECL library screening [199].

3.4 Undruggable targets and NGS

As mentioned above, an "Undruggable" target is a term given to sets of proteins that cannot be targeted by a specific treatment, yet they can be exploited for the development of treatments for various diseases.

Among these undruggable targets are non-enzymatic proteins, transcriptional factors, regulatory proteins, and scaffolding proteins [200, 201]. One such undruggable target is the Kristen Rat Sarcoma (KRAS) protein encoding a viral oncogene, detected in non-small cell lung cancer (NSCLC). Recently, KRAS mutations have been successfully targeted using different approaches, such as inhibition of downstream effectors, epigenomic approaches, post-translational modifications, and high-affinity KRAS binders, among others, wherein direct pharmacological inhibition of a *KRAS p.G12C* mutation is deemed possible, thus serving as an effective targeted treatment available for patients with advanced NSCLC [202]. Moreover, other members of the RAS family are deemed as undruggable targets in cancer, and several approaches have been used. Kato et al. have used NGS to evaluate the mutational status of 1937 patients with different cancers, and have observed that over 20% presented *RAS* alterations. Unfortunately, poor overall survival has been observed in spite of various treatment options that are offered; however, a better survival is observed for patients treated using a combined therapy targeting MAPK and non-MAPK pathways [203]. Among other undruggable targets, MYC and TP53 are known to have no enzymatic activities, and are located intracellularly. However, a Phase III trial is undergoing for TP53 using the APR-246 drug for myelodysplastic syndrome, and although there are no current clinical trials for MYC, an anti-MYC compound, OmoMYC, has been validated in multiple preclinical studies [204].

In other efforts, Zhou et al. have proposed the use of neoantigens, collected from patients with gastric cancer, for targeted therapies for gastric cancer disease [181]. In this study, six highly mutated genes along with high frequency HLA alleles have been identified, thus rendering neoantigens of these six genes as possible targets for immunotherapy of gastric cancer [205]. In another study on neuroblastoma, it is reported that a *MYCN* gene can be transformed into a druggable target by targeting different regulators of its pathway, such as β-estradiol and MAPK/ERK [206].

3.5 Drug resistance and NGS

Using NGS, a new gene was identified in *Acinetobacter baumannii* strain 863 conferring multi-drug resistance to this bacterial pathogen [207]. In another study, an antibiotic resistance signature of 25 genes was differentially expressed in *Staphylococcus aureus* [208]. Furthermore, it was reported that NGS might be successfully used for early identification of mutations related to drug resistance in transplant patients treated for cytomegalovirus [209].

In other studies, metagenomics NGS assays have been used to identify microbial composition and antibiotic resistance in water samples of Puget Sound (Washington State), and have reported that this could serve as a reliable protocol for providing accurate information on bacterial composition and antibiotic resistance in water samples [210]. Leprohon et al. have reviewed all critical information relevant to drug resistance and to resistance mechanism(s) in Leishmania infections generated from NGS analysis [211]. Furthermore, NGS has been successfully used for testing for HIV-1 drug resistance, although such studies are yet to be standardized [212–216]. Likewise, NGS and pyrosequencing have been used to investigate resistance of the *Influenta A* virus to baloxavir [217]. Moreover, NGS has also been used for detection of those *H. pylori* clones that are resistant to levofloxacin [218]. While RNA-seq data have been mined to identify novel fusion genes in gastrointestinal stromal tumor patients with resistance to imatinib [219].

4. DrugBank

Another important set of tools in drug discovery are the collective databases of drugs with detailed information about drugs, including their actions and targets. One such database is DrugBank, launched back in 2006, as it combines various resources offering clinical information, including chemical information about drugs and resources [220]. The main focus of DrugBank is to offer information relavent to mechanistic data, structures, and sequences about drugs and their targets. Furthermore, this resource is capable of providing tools for viewing, sorting, and searching both sequence and structure data [220]. Lately, DrugBank database has been further improved, as it now can offer information about 1467 FDA-approved drugs, 123 biotech drugs, 69 nutraceuticals, 4774 small molecule drugs, and 3116 experimental or unapproved drugs. There is also information related to withdrawn [57] and illicit [188] drugs. Furthermore, it has a higher drug target database for FDA-approved drugs, which includes 1565 non-redundant protein/DNA targets [221].

Due to its wealth of information, DrugBank has been used for a variety of drug applications, including target prediction [222], *in silico* discovery [223], metabolism prediction [224], docking or screening [225], as well as new uses of old drugs [226]. Additional applications are presented in **Table 3**.

Type of application	Drug tested	Disease	Reference(s)
Drug-target identification	Traditional Chinese medicine derived from *Trachelospermum jasminoides*	Rheumatoid arthritis	[227]
Molecular docking and simulation studies	Mitoxantrone, Leucovorin, Birinapant, and Dynasore	SARS-CoV-2 M ^{pro}	[228]
Virtual drug screening	Repositioning Dequalinium	hM_2 allosteric modulation	[229]
Drug metabolism prediction	Drugs related to P450 cytochrome enzymes	Seniors' Metabolism of Medications and Avoiding Adverse Drug Events	[230]
Drug screening/ discovery	All drugs correlated to viral proteins	SARS-CoV-2	[231]
Molecular docking, drug resistance	Carbapenems	*Acinetobacter baumannii* OXA class enzymes	[232]
Molecular docking, molecular dynamic simulation	Approve drug libraries for ACE2	SARS-CoV-2	[233]
In silico screening	Glycoprotein inhibitors	SARS-CoV-2	[234]
Drug repositioning	Drugs that target genes in pathways for treating depression	Treatment of resistant depression	[235]
Pharmacological analysis	JianPi Fu Recipe	Colon cancer LoVo cells metastasis	[236]
Multi regulatory pathways construction	Pivotal Drugs for pancreatic cancer	Pancreatic cancer	[237]
Drug repurposing	Drugs that inhibit proteases	SARS-CoV-2	[238, 239]
Drug repurposing		Hypertension	[240]
Pharmacological drug mechanism	Aloperine	Cardiovascular disease	[241]
Drug screening	Drugs targeting immune-related genes	Cervical cancer	[242]

Table 3.
Applications of the DrugBank database.

Although **Table 3** presents only a few studies employing the DrugBank database, a PubMed search for DrugBank has identified at least 505 published articles, from 2006 until 2020.

5. NGS in SARS-CoV-2 drug discovery

As infections with the SARS-CoV-2 virus have become more aggressive, there is an urgent need for evaluating different drugs that may contribute to a better and effective treatment of this infection. The majority of drugs used for SARS-CoV-2 treatment are drugs currently in use for treatment of other diseases [243–245], and these have been evaluated for their efficacy using computational drug discovery analysis [246–248].

Although NGS has been used primarily for genome identification of SARS-CoV-2 [249–252], as well as for evaluation of mutations developed during viral spread in different countries [253–255], there are some studies wherein RNA sequencing is used for identifying new drug treatments. One such study has used NGS for evaluation of affected genes during SARS-CoV-2 infections. In this study, different genes involved in RNA regulation, histone remodeling, cellular signaling, and chromatin remodeling are identified. Some of these identified genes have demonstrated either pro- or antiviral activities; thus, these genes could serve as potential tools for different therapies or vaccines [256]. In another study, a shotgun metatranscriptomics RNA sequencing technique is used for a cohort of New York SARS-CoV-2 infected patients, and have identified host-responses to SARS-CoV-2 infections in different pathways such as interferon, ACE, olfactory, and hematological pathways [179]. Moreover, they have also analyzed risks associated with angiotensin blockers and ACE inhibitor treatments in SARS-CoV-2 infected patients [179].

6. Features of microarrays and NGS and their relevance in drug discovery

In general, there are a variety of features for each of microarrays and NGS that render these platforms highly valuable in the arena of drug discovery and therapeutics, and these are summarized in **Table 4**.

Microarrays offer various advantages including expression analysis of cells or tissues at different states of disease, pharmacogenomics, toxicogenomics, and as well as for analysis and identification of SNPs. The microarray technology is useful for obtaining a good amount of information from small volume samples, and it is quite valuable for use in incorporating low-cost high-throughput assays in the drug discovery process. However, this technology has a number of disadvantages. These include high costs and long timelines, particularly related to re-design of microarray chips to include newly discovered genetic targets.

In comparison to microarrays, NGS offers more flexibility and higher cost-efficacy. In particular, this technology allows for identification of targets, screening of large numbers of compounds for use in therapeutics or treatments, as well as for identifying of unique biomarkers useful for discovery of new drug targets.

	Microarrays	**NGS**
Advantages	Expression of thousands of genes simultaneously; Low sample consumption; Easy sample preparation and control of experimental conditions; Data variability	High sensitivity; Quantitative; High dynamic range; No hybridization
Disadvantages	Competence required for data normalization and analysis; Limited dynamic range; Low sensitivity; Competitive hybridization	Complex sample preparation; Complex technology infrastructure required; High cost
Applications	Biomarker identification; Gene discovery; Vaccine development	Target identification; Compound screening; Biomarker identification; Drug resistance; Vaccine discovery

Table 4.
Benchmarks for NGS and microarrays in drug discovery.

7. Conclusions

Overall, although the word "limitation" still floats around, and with only 5% of novel molecular compounds are ultimately selected to enter the drug and therapeutic marketplace, new innovations in science and technology are critical in the arena of drug discovery and therapeutics. It is these ongoing research advances and technological innovations that will empower scientists to continue on in the pursuit of additional and more sophisticated, reliable, and efficient molecular tools, such as NGS and microarrays, that will be useful in the arena of drug discovery and therapeutics. These efforts, innovations, and technologies will undoubtedly continue to revolutionize the drug discovery industry that will aid in identifying better and more effective drugs, at much lower costs, and within shorter periods of time.

Funding

The funding for this book chapter is ensured by the PCCDI National Project: Genomic mapping of the population in the areas radioactively contaminated with heavy metals in order to increase national security- ARTEMIS.

Conflict of interest

The authors declare no conflict of interest.

Author details

Laura-Ancuta Pop[1], Oana Zanoaga[1], Paul Chiroi[1], Andreea Nutu[1], Schuyler S. Korban[2], Cristina Stefan[3,4], Alexandru Irimie[5] and Ioana Berindan-Neagoe[1*]

1 Research Center for Functional Genomics, Biomedicine and Translational Medicine, Iuliu Hatieganu University of Medicine and Pharmacy, Cluj-Napoca, Romania

2 Department of Natural Resources and Environmental Sciences, University of Illinois at Urbana-Champaign, Urbana, Illinois, USA

3 SingHealth Duke-NUS Global Health Institute (SDGHI), Duke-NUS Medical School, Singapore

4 African Medical Research and Innovation Institute, Cape Town, South Africa

5 Department of Surgical Oncology and Gynecological Oncology, University of Medicine and Pharmacy Iuliu Hatieganu, Cluj-Napoca, Romania

*Address all correspondence to: ioananeagoe29@gmail.com

References

[1] Doroshow JH, Kummar S. Translational research in oncology--10 years of progress and future prospects. Replace with: Nat. Rev. Clin. Oncol. 2014;11(11):649-62.

[2] Kunnumakkara AB, Bordoloi D, Sailo BL, Roy NK, Thakur KK, Banik K, et al. Cancer drug development: The missing links. Exp. Biol. Med. 2019;244(8):663-89.

[3] Wilding JL, Bodmer WF. Cancer cell lines for drug discovery and development. Cancer Res. 2014; 74(9):2377-84.

[4] Roy PS, Saikia BJ. Cancer and cure: A critical analysis. Indian J. Cancer. 2016;53(3):441-2.

[5] Bordoloi D, Sailo, B.L., Manteghi, N., Padmavathi, G., Kunnumakkara, A.B. Introduction and basic concepts of cancer. Cancer Cell Chemoresist. Chemosensit. 2018.

[6] Bray F, Ferlay J, Soerjomataram I, Siegel RL, Torre LA, Jemal A. Global cancer statistics 2018: GLOBOCAN estimates of incidence and mortality worldwide for 36 cancers in 185 countries. CA: Cancer J. Clin. 2018; 68(6):394-424.

[7] Ferlay J, Colombet M, Soerjomataram I, Mathers C, Parkin DM, Piñeros M, et al. Estimating the global cancer incidence and mortality in 2018: GLOBOCAN sources and methods. Int. J. Cancer. 2019; 144(8):1941-53.

[8] Vasan N, Baselga J, Hyman DM. A view on drug resistance in cancer. Nature. 2019;575(7782):299-309.

[9] Eder J, Herrling PL. Trends in Modern Drug Discovery. Handbook of Exp. Pharmacol. 2016;232:3-22.

[10] Li JW, Vederas JC. Drug discovery and natural products: end of an era or an endless frontier? Science. 2009; 325(5937):161-5.

[11] Chan HCS, Shan H, Dahoun T, Vogel H, Yuan S. Advancing Drug Discovery via Artificial Intelligence. Trends Pharmacol. Sci. 2019;40(8): 592-604.

[12] Overington JP, Al-Lazikani B, Hopkins AL. How many drug targets are there? Nat. Rev. Drug Discov. 2006; 5(12):993-6.

[13] Adams CP, Brantner VV. Estimating the cost of new drug development: is it really 802 million dollars? Health affairs. 2006;25(2):420-8.

[14] Mariotto AB, Enewold L, Zhao J, Zeruto CA, Yabroff KR. Medical Care Costs Associated with Cancer Survivorship in the United States. Cancer Epidemiol Biomarkers Prev. 2020 Jul;29(7):1304-1312.

[15] Prasad S, Gupta SC, Aggarwal BB. Serendipity in Cancer Drug Discovery: Rational or Coincidence? Trends Pharmacol. Sci.. 2016;37(6):435-50.

[16] Workman P, Antolin AA, Al-Lazikani B. Transforming cancer drug discovery with Big Data and AI. Expert Opin Drug Discov. 2019; 14(11):1089-95.

[17] Garon EB, Rizvi NA, Hui R, Leighl N, Balmanoukian AS, Eder JP, et al. Pembrolizumab for the treatment of non-small-cell lung cancer. New England J. Med. 2015;372(21):2018-28.

[18] Gyawali B, Hwang TJ, Vokinger KN, Booth CM, Amir E, Tibau A. Patient-Centered Cancer Drug Development: Clinical Trials, Regulatory Approval, and Value Assessment. American Society of Clinical Oncology educational book

American Society of Clinical Oncology Annual Meeting. 2019;39:374-87.

[19] Arshad Z, Smith J, Roberts M, Lee WH, Davies B, Bure K, et al. Open Access Could Transform Drug Discovery: A Case Study of JQ1. Expert Opin. Drug Discov. 2016;11(3):321-32.

[20] Di Resta C, Galbiati S, Carrera P, Ferrari M. Next-generation sequencing approach for the diagnosis of human diseases: open challenges and new opportunities. Ejifcc. 2018;29(1):4-14.

[21] Yadav NK, Shukla P, Omer A, Pareek S, Srivastava AK, Bansode FW, et al. Next generation sequencing: potential and application in drug discovery. Scient. World J. 2014;2014:802437.

[22] Loewe RP, Nelson PJ. Microarray bioinformatics. Methods Mol. Biol. 2011;671:295-320.

[23] Carrara L, Lavezzi SM, Borella E, De Nicolao G, Magni P, Poggesi I. Current mathematical models for cancer drug discovery. Expert Opin. Drug Discov. 2017;12(8):785-99.

[24] Dong J, Bao J, Feng R, Zhao Z, Lu Q, Wang G, et al. Circulating microRNAs: a novel potential biomarker for diagnosing acute aortic dissection. Scient. Rep. 2017;7(1):12784.

[25] Shukla AK, Tripathi D. Identification of potential biomarkers on microarray data using distributed gene selection approach. Math. Biosci. 2019;315:108230.

[26] Tikhonov A, Smoldovskaya O, Feyzkhanova G, Kushlinskii N, Rubina A. Glycan-specific antibodies as potential cancer biomarkers: a focus on microarray applications. Clin. Chem. Lab. Med. 2020;58(10):1611-22.

[27] Duan S, Gong B, Wang P, Huang H, Luo L, Liu F. Novel prognostic biomarkers of gastric cancer based on gene expression microarray: COL12A1, GSTA3, FGA and FGG. Mol. Med. Rep. 2018;18(4):3727-36.

[28] Ciocan-Cartita CA, Jurj A, Zanoaga O, Cojocneanu R, Pop LA, Moldovan A, et al. New insights in gene expression alteration as effect of doxorubicin drug resistance in triple negative breast cancer cells. J. Exp. Clin. Cancer Res. 2020;39(1):241.

[29] Lajos R, Braicu C, Jurj A, Chira S, Cojocneanu-Petric R, Pileczki V, et al. A miRNAs profile evolution of triple negative breast cancer cells in the presence of a possible adjuvant therapy and senescence inducer. J. BUON 2018;23(3):692-705.

[30] Chen J, Goodchild TT, Brott BC, Li J, King SB, 3rd, Chronos N, et al. Microarray applications in occlusive vascular disease. Cardiovas. Hematol. Agents Med. Chem. 2011;9(2):84-94.

[31] Yoo SM, Choi JH, Lee SY, Yoo NC. Applications of DNA microarray in disease diagnostics. J. Microbiol. Biotech. 2009;19(7):635-46.

[32] Marzancola MG, Sedighi A, Li PC. DNA Microarray-Based Diagnostics. Methods Mol. Biol. 2016;1368:161-78.

[33] Patel A, Cheung SW. Application of DNA Microarray to Clinical Diagnostics. Methods Mol. Boil. 2016;1368:111-32.

[34] Ling H, Pickard K, Ivan C, Isella C, Ikuo M, Mitter R, et al. The clinical and biological significance of MIR-224 expression in colorectal cancer metastasis. Gut. 2016;65(6):977-89.

[35] Pease AC, Solas D, Sullivan EJ, Cronin MT, Holmes CP, Fodor SP. Light-generated oligonucleotide arrays for rapid DNA sequence analysis. Proc. Natl. Acad. Sci. U.S.A. 1994;91(11): 5022-6.

[36] Held GA, Grinstein G, Tu Y. Relationship between gene expression

and observed intensities in DNA microarrays--a modeling study. Nucleic Acids Res. 2006;34(9):e70.

[37] Oberthuer A, Juraeva D, Li L, Kahlert Y, Westermann F, Eils R, et al. Comparison of performance of one-color and two-color gene-expression analyses in predicting clinical endpoints of neuroblastoma patients. Pharmacog. J. 2010;10(4):258-66.

[38] Rando O. Nucleic Acid Platform Technologies. Cold Spring Harbor protocols. 2019;2019(9).

[39] Hardiman G. Microarray platforms--comparisons and contrasts. Pharmacogenomics. 2004;5(5):487-502.

[40] Miller MB, Tang YW. Basic concepts of microarrays and potential applications in clinical microbiology. Clin. Microbiol. Rev. 2009;22(4):611-33.

[41] Grist SM, Nasseri SS, Poon T, Roskelley C, Cheung KC. On-chip clearing of arrays of 3-D cell cultures and micro-tissues. Biomicrofluidics. 2016;10(4):044107.

[42] Bovard D, Sandoz A, Luettich K, Frentzel S, Iskandar A, Marescotti D, et al. A lung/liver-on-a-chip platform for acute and chronic toxicity studies. Lab on a chip. 2018;18(24):3814-29.

[43] Bumgarner R. Overview of DNA microarrays: types, applications, and their future. Curr. Protocol. Mol. Biol. 2013;Chapter 22:Unit 22.1.

[44] Zhao S, Niu F, Xu CY, Ye L, Bi GB, Chen L, et al. Microarray and ChIP-seq data analysis revealed changes in p53-mediated transcriptional regulation in Nutlin-3-treated U2OS cells. Mol. Med. Rep. 2015;12(3):4284-90.

[45] Johnston M. Gene chips: array of hope for understanding gene regulation. Curr. Boil: CB. 1998;8(5):R171-4.

[46] Chira S, Raduly L, Braicu C, Jurj A, Cojocneanu-Petric R, Pop L, et al. Premature senescence activation in DLD-1 colorectal cancer cells through adjuvant therapy to induce a miRNA profile modulating cellular death. Exp. Therap. Med. 2018;16(2):1241-9.

[47] Le KQ, Prabhakar BS, Hong WJ, Li LC. Alternative splicing as a biomarker and potential target for drug discovery. Acta Pharmacol. Sinica. 2015;36(10):1212-8.

[48] Leibrand CR, Price DK, Figg WD. Androgen receptor splice variant 7 (AR-V7) and drug efficacy in castration-resistant prostate cancer: Biomarker for treatment selection exclusion or inclusion? Cancer Biol. Therapy. 2016;17(5):467-9.

[49] Zhang T, Karsh LI, Nissenblatt MJ, Canfield SE. Androgen Receptor Splice Variant, AR-V7, as a Biomarker of Resistance to Androgen Axis-Targeted Therapies in Advanced Prostate Cancer. Clin. Genitourinary Cancer. 2020; 18(1):1-10.

[50] Huang C-W, Lin Y-T, Ding S-T, Lo L-L, Wang P-H, Lin E-C, et al. Efficient SNP Discovery by Combining Microarray and Lab-on-a-Chip Data for Animal Breeding and Selection. Microarrays. 2015;4(4):570-95.

[51] Ji Y, Mishra RK, Davuluri RV. In silico analysis of alternative splicing on drug-target gene interactions. Sci. Rep. 2020;10(1):134.

[52] Cojocneanu R, Braicu C, Raduly L, Jurj A, Zanoaga O, Magdo L, et al. Plasma and Tissue Specific miRNA Expression Pattern and Functional Analysis Associated to Colorectal Cancer Patients. Cancers. 2020;12(4).

[53] Finan C, Gaulton A, Kruger FA, Lumbers RT, Shah T, Engmann J, et al. The druggable genome and support for target identification and validation in

drug development. Science Translat. Med. 2017;9(383).

[54] Roden DM, McLeod HL, Relling MV, Williams MS, Mensah GA, Peterson JF, et al. Pharmacogenomics. Lancet. 2019; 394(10197):521-32.

[55] Baldwin DA, Sarnowski CP, Reddy SA, Blair IA, Clapper M, Lazarus P, et al. Development of a genotyping microarray for studying the role of gene-environment interactions in risk for lung cancer. J Biomol Tech. 2013;24(4):198-217.

[56] Dally S, Lemuth K, Kaase M, Rupp S, Knabbe C, Weile J. DNA microarray for genotyping antibiotic resistance determinants in Acinetobacter baumannii clinical isolates. Antimicrob Agents Chemother. 2013;57(10):4761-8.

[57] Neverov AA, Riddell MA, Moss WJ, Volokhov DV, Rota PA, Lowe LE, et al. Genotyping of measles virus in clinical specimens on the basis of oligonucleotide microarray hybridization patterns. J Clin Microbiol. 2006;44(10):3752-9.

[58] Shinawi M, Cheung SW. The array CGH and its clinical applications. Drug Discov. Today. 2008;13(17-18):760-70.

[59] Bejjani BA, Shaffer LG. Application of array-based comparative genomic hybridization to clinical diagnostics. The Journal of molecular diagnostics : J. Mol. Diagnost. 2006;8(5):528-33.

[60] Yang HL, Zhu YZ, Qin JH, He P, Jiang XC, Zhao GP, et al. In silico and microarray-based genomic approaches to identifying potential vaccine candidates against *Leptospira interrogans*. BMC Genomics. 2006;7:293.

[61] Hindson BJ, Ness KD, Masquelier DA, Belgrader P, Heredia NJ, Makarewicz AJ, et al. High-throughput droplet digital PCR system for absolute quantitation of DNA copy number. Anal. Chem. 2011;83(22):8604-10.

[62] Hindson CM, Chevillet JR, Briggs HA, Gallichotte EN, Ruf IK, Hindson BJ, et al. Absolute quantification by droplet digital PCR versus analog real-time PCR. Nat. Methods. 2013;10(10):1003-5.

[63] Galbiati S, Damin F, Ferraro L, Soriani N, Burgio V, Ronzoni M, et al. Microarray Approach Combined with ddPCR: An Useful Pipeline for the Detection and Quantification of Circulating Tumour dna Mutations. Cells. 2019;8(8).

[64] Gelsomino L, Gu G, Rechoum Y, Beyer AR, Pejerrey SM, Tsimelzon A, et al. ESR1 mutations affect anti-proliferative responses to tamoxifen through enhanced cross-talk with IGF signaling. Breast Cancer Res. Treat. 2016;157(2):253-65.

[65] Sivarajah S, Kostiuk M, Lindsay C, Puttagunta L, O'Connell DA, Harris J, et al. EGFR as a biomarker of smoking status and survival in oropharyngeal squamous cell carcinoma. J. Otolaryngol. 2019;48(1):1.

[66] Hall SM, Coulter SJ, Knudsen GA, Sanders JM, Birnbaum LS. Gene expression changes in immune response pathways following oral administration of tetrabromobisphenol A (TBBPA) in female Wistar Han rats. Toxicol. Lett. 2017;272:68-74.

[67] Vejdovszky K, Sack M, Jarolim K, Aichinger G, Somoza MM, Marko D. In vitro combinatory effects of the Alternaria mycotoxins alternariol and altertoxin II and potentially involved miRNAs. Toxicol. Lett. 2017; 267:45-52.

[68] Cho SY, Oh Y, Jeong EM, Park S, Lee D, Wang X, et al. Amplification of transglutaminase 2 enhances tumor-promoting inflammation in gastric cancers. Exp. Mol. Med. 2020;52(5): 854-64.

[69] Dang CV, Reddy EP, Shokat KM, Soucek L. Drugging the 'undruggable' cancer targets. Nat. Rev. Cancer. 2017;17(8):502-8.

[70] Ray D, Cuneo KC, Rehemtulla A, Lawrence TS, Nyati MK. Inducing Oncoprotein Degradation to Improve Targeted Cancer Therapy. Neoplasia (New York, NY). 2015;17(9):697-703.

[71] Hallin J, Engstrom LD, Hargis L, Calinisan A, Aranda R, Briere DM, et al. The KRAS(G12C) Inhibitor MRTX849 Provides Insight toward Therapeutic Susceptibility of KRAS-Mutant Cancers in Mouse Models and Patients. Cancer discovery. 2020;10(1):54-71.

[72] Cox AD, Fesik SW, Kimmelman AC, Luo J, Der CJ. Drugging the undruggable RAS: Mission possible? Nat. Rev. Drug Discovery. 2014;13(11):828-51.

[73] Moore AR, Rosenberg SC, McCormick F, Malek S. RAS-targeted therapies: is the undruggable drugged? Nat. Rev. Drug Discovery. 2020; 19(8):533-52.

[74] Allen-Petersen BL, Sears RC. Mission Possible: Advances in MYC Therapeutic Targeting in Cancer. BioDrugs. 2019; 33(5):539-53.

[75] Duffy MJ, Synnott NC, Crown J. Mutant p53 as a target for cancer treatment. Eur. J. Cancer. 2017;83: 258-65.

[76] Zhang D, Zhang G, Hu X, Wu L, Feng Y, He S, et al. Oncogenic RAS Regulates Long Noncoding RNA Orilnc1 in Human Cancer. Cancer Res. 2017; 77(14):3745-57.

[77] Tao J, Zhang R, Singh S, Poddar M, Xu E, Oertel M, et al. Targeting β-catenin in hepatocellular cancers induced by coexpression of mutant β-catenin and K-Ras in mice. Hepatology. 2017;65(5):1581-99.

[78] Kant R, Yen CH, Hung JH, Lu CK, Tung CY, Chang PC, et al. Induction of GNMT by 1,2,3,4,6-penta-O-galloyl-beta-D-glucopyranoside through proteasome-independent MYC downregulation in hepatocellular carcinoma. Scient. Rep. 2019;9(1):1968.

[79] Ye L, Pan J, Liang M, Pasha MA, Shen X, D'Souza SS, et al. A critical role for c-Myc in group 2 innate lymphoid cell activation. Allergy. 2020;75(4):841-52.

[80] Xu J, Chen Y, Huo D, Khramtsov A, Khramtsova G, Zhang C, et al. β-catenin regulates c-Myc and CDKN1A expression in breast cancer cells. Molecular carcinogenesis. 2016;55(5):431-9.

[81] Charni M, Molchadsky A, Goldstein I, Solomon H, Tal P, Goldfinger N, et al. Novel p53 target genes secreted by the liver are involved in non-cell-autonomous regulation. Cell Death Diff. 2016;23(3):509-20.

[82] Koyama R, Tamura M, Nakagaki T, Ohashi T, Idogawa M, Suzuki H, et al. Identification and characterization of a metastatic suppressor BRMS1L as a target gene of p53. Cancer Sci. 2017;108(12):2413-21.

[83] Lee CH, Macgregor PF. Using microarrays to predict resistance to chemotherapy in cancer patients. Pharmacogenomics. 2004;5(6):611-25.

[84] Xu C, Yu Y, Ding F. Microarray analysis of circular RNA expression profiles associated with gemcitabine resistance in pancreatic cancer cells. Oncol. Rep. 2018;40(1):395-404.

[85] Lu L, Wu M, Lu Y, Zhao Z, Liu T, Fu W, et al. MicroRNA-424 regulates cisplatin resistance of gastric cancer by targeting SMURF1 based on GEO database and primary validation in human gastric cancer tissues. Oncol. Targ. Therapy. 2019;12:7623-36.

[86] Januchowski R, Zawierucha P, Ruciński M, Zabel M. Microarray-based

detection and expression analysis of extracellular matrix proteins in drug-resistant ovarian cancer cell lines. Oncology Rep. 2014;32(5):1981-90.

[87] Januchowski R, Sterzyńska K, Zawierucha P, Ruciński M, Świerczewska M, Partyka M, et al. Microarray-based detection and expression analysis of new genes associated with drug resistance in ovarian cancer cell lines. Oncotarget. 2017;8(30):49944-58.

[88] Jurj A, Pop LA, Zanoaga O, Ciocan-Cârtiță CA, Cojocneanu R, Moldovan C, et al. New Insights in Gene Expression Alteration as Effect of Paclitaxel Drug Resistance in Triple Negative Breast Cancer Cells. Cellular Physiol. Biochem. 2020;54(4):648-64.

[89] You S, Gao L. Identification of NMU as a potential gene conferring alectinib resistance in non-small cell lung cancer based on bioinformatics analyses. Gene. 2018;678:137-42.

[90] Vert A, Castro J, Ribó M, Vilanova M, Benito A. Transcriptional profiling of NCI/ADR-RES cells unveils a complex network of signaling pathways and molecular mechanisms of drug resistance. OncoTargets Therapy. 2018;11:221-37.

[91] Tovar V, Cornella H, Moeini A, Vidal S, Hoshida Y, Sia D, et al. Tumour initiating cells and IGF/FGF signalling contribute to sorafenib resistance in hepatocellular carcinoma. Gut. 2017; 66(3):530-40.

[92] Card R, Zhang J, Das P, Cook C, Woodford N, Anjum MF. Evaluation of an expanded microarray for detecting antibiotic resistance genes in a broad range of gram-negative bacterial pathogens. Antimicrobial Agents Chemother. 2013;57(1):458-65.

[93] Frye JG, Lindsey RL, Rondeau G, Porwollik S, Long F, McClelland M, et al. Development of a DNA microarray to detect antimicrobial resistance genes identified in the National Center for Biotechnology Information database. Microbial Drug Resist. 2010;16(1):9-19.

[94] Song Y, Dou F, Zhou Z, Yang N, Zhong J, Pan J, et al. Microarray-Based Detection and Clinical Evaluation for Helicobacter pylori Resistance to Clarithromycin or Levofloxacin and the Genotype of CYP2C19 in 1083 Patients. BioMed Res. Intl. 2018;2018:2684836.

[95] Azizi M, Zaferani M, Dogan B, Zhang S, Simpson KW, Abbaspourrad A. Nanoliter-Sized Microchamber/Microarray Microfluidic Platform for Antibiotic Susceptibility Testing. Anal. Chem. 2018;90(24):14137-44.

[96] Charnock C, Samuelsen Ø, Nordlie AL, Hjeltnes B. Use of a Commercially Available Microarray to Characterize Antibiotic-Resistant Clinical Isolates of *Klebsiella pneumoniae*. Current Microbiol. 2018;75(2):163-72.

[97] Abulwerdi FA, Xu W, Ageeli AA, Yonkunas MJ, Arun G, Nam H, et al. Selective Small-Molecule Targeting of a Triple Helix Encoded by the Long Noncoding RNA, MALAT1. ACS Chem. Biol. 2019;14(2):223-35.

[98] Ursu A, Vézina-Dawod S, Disney MD. Methods to identify and optimize small molecules interacting with RNA (SMIRNAs). Drug Discov. Today. 2019;24(10):2002-16.

[99] Hafeez H, Laurent K, Xiaohui L, Gogce C, Jonas B, Daniel A, et al. Design of a Small Molecule That Stimulates VEGFA Informed from an Expanded Encyclopedia of RNA Fold-Small Molecule Interactions Add - ChemRxiv.

[100] Xu F, Wu J, Wang S, Durmus NG, Gurkan UA, Demirci U. Micro-engineering methods for cell-based microarrays and high-throughput

drug-screening applications. Biofabrication. 2011;3(3):034101.

[101] Bailey SN, Sabatini DM, Stockwell BR. Microarrays of small molecules embedded in biodegradable polymers for use in mammalian cell-based screens. Proc. Natl. Acad. Sci. U.S.A. 2004;101(46):16144-9.

[102] Mateen R, Ali MM, Hoare T. A printable hydrogel microarray for drug screening avoids false positives associated with promiscuous aggregating inhibitors. Nat. Commun. 2018;9(1):602.

[103] Ooko E, Saeed ME, Kadioglu O, Sarvi S, Colak M, Elmasaoudi K, et al. Artemisinin derivatives induce iron-dependent cell death (ferroptosis) in tumor cells. Phytomedicine. 2015;22(11): 1045-54.

[104] Liao P, Li W, Liu R, Teer JK, Xu B, Zhang W, et al. Genome-scale analysis identifies SERPINE1 and SPARC as diagnostic and prognostic biomarkers in gastric cancer. OncoTargets Therapy. 2018;11:6969-80.

[105] Sco EJ, Saeed M, Law BY, Wu AG, Kadioglu O, Greten HJ, et al. Pharmacogenomics of Scopoletin in Tumor Cells. Molecules (Basel, Switzerland). 2016;21(4):496.

[106] Zhu QN, Renaud H, Guo Y. Bioinformatics-based identification of miR-542-5p as a predictive biomarker in breast cancer therapy. Hereditas. 2018; 155:17.

[107] Gao YF, Zhu T, Mao CX, Liu ZX, Wang ZB, Mao XY, et al. PPIC, EMP3 and CHI3L1 Are Novel Prognostic Markers for High Grade Glioma. Int. J. Mol. Sci. 2016;17(11).

[108] Zambrano T, Hirata RDC, Hirata MH, Cerda Á, Salazar LA. Altered microRNome Profiling in Statin-Induced HepG2 Cells: A Pilot Study Identifying Potential new Biomarkers Involved in Lipid-Lowering Treatment. Cardiov. Drugs Therapy. 2015;29(6):509-18.

[109] Fujita K, Nonomura N. Urinary biomarkers of prostate cancer. Int. J. Urology. 2018;25(9):770-9.

[110] Wu J, Wheeldon I, Guo Y, Lu T, Du Y, Wang B, et al. A sandwiched microarray platform for benchtop cell-based high throughput screening. Biomaterials. 2011;32(3):841-8.

[111] Dalerba P, Sahoo D, Paik S, Guo X, Yothers G, Song N, et al. CDX2 as a Prognostic Biomarker in Stage II and Stage III Colon Cancer. The New England journal of medicine. 2016;374(3):211-22.

[112] Lin C, Zhang S, Wang Y, Wang Y, Nice E, Guo C, et al. Functional Role of a Novel Long Noncoding RNA TTN-AS1 in Esophageal Squamous Cell Carcinoma Progression and Metastasis. Clin. Cancer Res. 2018;24(2):486-98.

[113] Carstens MR, Fisher RC, Acharya AP, Butterworth EA, Scott E, Huang EH, et al. Drug-eluting microarrays to identify effective chemotherapeutic combinations targeting patient-derived cancer stem cells. Proc. Natl. Acad. Sci. U.S.A. 2015;112(28):8732-7.

[114] Ding CH, Yin C, Chen SJ, Wen LZ, Ding K, Lei SJ, et al. The HNF1α-regulated lncRNA HNF1A-AS1 reverses the malignancy of hepatocellular carcinoma by enhancing the phosphatase activity of SHP-1. Mol. Cancer. 2018;17(1):63.

[115] Kudou M, Shiozaki A, Yamazato Y, Katsurahara K, Kosuga T, Shoda K, et al. The expression and role of TRPV2 in esophageal squamous cell carcinoma. Sci. Rep. 2019;9(1):16055.

[116] Na Z, Pan S, Uttamchandani M, Yao SQ. Protein-Protein Interaction Inhibitors of BRCA1 Discovered Using

Small Molecule Microarrays. Methods Mol. Biol. 2017;1518:139-56.

[117] Lin LC, Kuo TT, Chang HY, Liu WS, Hsia SM, Huang TC. Manzamine A Exerts Anticancer Activity against Human Colorectal Cancer Cells. Marine drugs. 2018;16(8).

[118] Li L, Gao R, Yu Y, Kaul Z, Wang J, Kalra RS, et al. Tumor suppressor activity of miR-451: Identification of CARF as a new target. Sci. Rep. 2018; 8(1):375.

[119] Sriram K, Wiley SZ, Moyung K, Gorr MW, Salmerón C, Marucut J, et al. Detection and Quantification of GPCR mRNA: An Assessment and Implications of Data from High-Content Methods. ACS omega. 2019;4(16):17048-59.

[120] Zhao B, Zhao Y, Sun Y, Niu H, Sheng L, Huang D, et al. Alterations in mRNA profiles of trastuzumab-resistant Her-2-positive breast cancer. Mol. Med. Rep. 2018;18(1):139-46.

[121] Zhou Y, Zou H, Yau C, Zhao L, Hall SC, Drummond DC, et al. Discovery of internalizing antibodies to basal breast cancer cells. Protein Eng. Design Sel. 2018;31(1):17-28.

[122] Qu T, Li YP, Li XH, Chen Y. Identification of potential biomarkers and drugs for papillary thyroid cancer based on gene expression profile analysis. Mol. Med. Rep. 2016;14(6): 5041-8.

[123] Nguyen MT, Ho-Huynh TD. Nam Dia long, a Vietnamese folk formula, induces apoptosis in MCF-7 cells through various mechanisms of action. BMC Complem. Alt. Med. 2017;17(1): 522.

[124] Yang PM, Lin LS, Liu TP. Sorafenib Inhibits Ribonucleotide Reductase Regulatory Subunit M2 (RRM2) in Hepatocellular Carcinoma Cells. Biomolecules. 2020;10(1).

[125] Chen CH, Liu YM, Pan SL, Liu YR, Liou JP, Yen Y. Trichlorobenzene-substituted azaaryl compounds as novel FGFR inhibitors exhibiting potent antitumor activity in bladder cancer cells in vitro and in vivo. Oncotarget. 2016;7(18):26374-87.

[126] Ayyar VS, Sukumaran S, DuBois DC, Almon RR, Jusko WJ. Modeling Corticosteroid Pharmacogenomics and Proteomics in Rat Liver. J. Pharm. Exp. Therap. 2018;367(1):168-83.

[127] Hongkaew Y, Medhasi S, Pasomsub E, Ngamsamut N, Puangpetch A, Vanwong N, et al. UGT1A1 polymorphisms associated with prolactin response in risperidone-treated children and adolescents with autism spectrum disorder. Pharmaco-genomics J. 2018;18(6):740-8.

[128] Eugene AR, Masiak J, Eugene B. Predicting lithium treatment response in bipolar patients using gender-specific gene expression biomarkers and machine learning. F1000Research. 2018;7:474.

[129] Faiz A, Donovan C, Nieuwenhuis MA, van den Berge M, Postma DS, Yao S, et al. Latrophilin receptors: novel bronchodilator targets in asthma. Thorax. 2017;72(1):74-82.

[130] Katsuma S, Tsujimoto G. Genome medicine promised by microarray technology. Expert Rev. Mol. Diagno. 2001;1(4):377-82.

[131] Lamb J, Crawford ED, Peck D, Modell JW, Blat IC, Wrobel MJ, et al. The Connectivity Map: using gene-expression signatures to connect small molecules, genes, and disease. Science. 2006;313(5795):1929-35.

[132] Xiong Y, Walker K, Min X, Hale C, Tran T, Komorowski R, et al. Long-acting MIC-1/GDF15 molecules to treat obesity: Evidence from mice to monkeys. Science Transl. Med. 2017;9(412).

[133] Greetham D, Lappin DF, Rajendran R, O'Donnell L, Sherry L, Ramage G, et al. The application of phenotypic microarray analysis to anti-fungal drug development. J. Microbiol. Methods. 2017;134:35-7.

[134] Broszeit F, Tzarum N, Zhu X, Nemanichvili N, Eggink D, Leenders T, et al. N-Glycolylneuraminic Acid as a Receptor for Influenza A Viruses. Cell Rep. 2019;27(11):3284-94.e6.

[135] Stencel-Baerenwald JE, Reiss K, Reiter DM, Stehle T, Dermody TS. The sweet spot: defining virus-sialic acid interactions. Nat. Rev. Microbiol. 2014;12(11):739-49.

[136] Li O, Geng X, Ma Q, Wang W, Liu R, Yin Z, et al. Gene Microarray Integrated with High-Throughput Proteomics for the Discovery of Transthyretin in Rhabdomyolysis-Induced Acute Kidney Injury. Cell. Physiol. Biochem. 2017;43(4):1673-88.

[137] Wilk G, Braun R. regQTLs: Single nucleotide polymorphisms that modulate microRNA regulation of gene expression in tumors. PLoS Genet. 2018;14(12):e1007837.

[138] Hiono T, Matsuda A, Wagatsuma T, Okamatsu M, Sakoda Y, Kuno A. Lectin microarray analyses reveal host cell-specific glycan profiles of the hema-gglutinins of influenza A viruses. Virology. 2019;527:132-40.

[139] Sabalza M, Barber CA, Abrams WR, Montagna R, Malamud D. Zika Virus Specific Diagnostic Epitope Discovery. J. Visual. Exp. 2017(130).

[140] Ma C, Lv Q, Teng S, Yu Y, Niu K, Yi C. Identifying key genes in rheumatoid arthritis by weighted gene co-expression network analysis. Int. J. Rheumatic Dis. 2017;20(8):971-9.

[141] Song J, Kim D, Hong J, Kim GW, Jung J, Park S, et al. Meta-Analysis of Polymyositis and Dermatomyositis Microarray Data Reveals Novel Genetic Biomarkers. Genes. 2019;10(11).

[142] Yang PM, Hong YH, Hsu KC, Liu TP. p38α/S1P/SREBP2 activation by the SAM-competitive EZH2 inhibitor GSK343 limits its anticancer activity but creates a druggable vulnerability in hepatocellular carcinoma. Amer. J. Cancer Res. 2019; 9(10):2120-39.

[143] Muhammad SA, Raza W, Nguyen T, Bai B, Wu X, Chen J. Cellular Signaling Pathways in Insulin Resistance-Systems Biology Analyses of Microarray Dataset Reveals New Drug Target Gene Signatures of Type 2 Diabetes Mellitus. Front. Physiol. 2017;8:13.

[144] Elmessaoudi-Idrissi M, Windisch MP, Kettani A, Altawalah H, Pineau P, Benjelloun S, et al. An Integrative Gene Expression Microarray Meta-analysis Identifies Host Factors and Key Signatures Involved in Hepatitis B Virus Infection. Infect. Disord. Drug Targ. 2020;20(5):698-707.

[145] Rabinowitz JA, Lainson JC, Johnston SA, Dichnelt CW. Non-natural amino acid peptide microarrays to discover Ebola virus glycoprotein ligands. Chem. Commun. 2018;54(12):1417-20.

[146] Kusi-Appiah AE, Lowry TW, Darrow EM, Wilson KA, Chadwick BP, Davidson MW, et al. Quantitative dose-response curves from subcellular lipid multilayer microarrays. Lab on a chip. 2015;15(16):3397-404.

[147] Fu J. Microarray Selection of Cooperative Peptides for Modulating Enzyme Activities. Microarrays. 2017;6(2).

[148] Pateisky P, Pils D, Szabo L, Kuessel L, Husslein H, Schmitz A, et al. hsav-miRNA-154-5p expression in plasma of endometriosis patients is a potential diagnostic marker for the disease. Reproduct. Biomed. Online. 2018;37(4):449-66.

[149] Jia X, Yu H, Zhang H, Si Y, Tian D, Zhao X, et al. Integrated analysis of different microarray studies to identify candidate genes in type 1 diabetes. J. Diabetes. 2017;9(2):149-57.

[150] Yen CC, Chen SC, Hung GY, Wu PK, Chua WY, Lin YC, et al. Expression profile-driven discovery of AURKA as a treatment target for liposarcoma. Int. J. Oncol. 2019;55(4): 938-48.

[151] Bi BL, Wang HJ, Bian H, Tian ZT. Identification of therapeutic targets of ischemic stroke with DNA microarray. Eur. Rev. Med. Pharmacol. 2015;19(21): 4012-9.

[152] Bae N, Viviano M, Su X, Lv J, Cheng D, Sagum C, et al. Developing Spindlin1 small-molecule inhibitors by using protein microarrays. Nat. Chem. Biol. 2017;13(7):750-6.

[153] Nguyen BN, Okuno Y, Ajiro M, Iida K, Denawa M, Yamamoto M, et al. Retinoid derivative Tp80 exhibits anti-hepatitis C virus activity through restoration of GI-GPx expression. J. Med. Virol. 2017;89(7):1224-34.

[154] Zlotkowski K, Hewitt WM, Sinniah RS, Tropea JE, Needle D, Lountos GT, et al. A Small-Molecule Microarray Approach for the Identification of E2 Enzyme Inhibitors in Ubiquitin-Like Conjugation Pathways. SLAS Discov. 2017;22(6): 760-6.

[155] Sun AG, Lin AQ, Huang SY, Huo D, Cong CH. Identification of potential drugs for Parkinson's disease based on a sub-pathway method. Int. J. Neurosc. 2016;126(4):318-25.

[156] Sun K, Xie Z, Wang J, Ling M, Li Y, Qiu C. Bioinformatics-based study to detect chemical compounds that show potential as treatments for pulmonary thromboembolism. Int. J. Mol. Med. 2019;43(1):276-84.

[157] Jiang H, Wu FR, Liu J, Qin XJ, Jiang NN, Li WP. Effect of astragalosides on long non-coding RNA expression profiles in rats with adjuvant-induced arthritis. Int. J. Mol. Med. 2019;44(4): 1344-56.

[158] Yoshinaga T, Uwabe K, Naito S, Higashino K, Nakano T, Numata Y, et al. AM251 Suppresses Epithelial-Mesenchymal Transition of Renal Tubular Epithelial Cells. PloS one. 2016; 11(12):e0167848.

[159] Iwanowycz S, Wang J, Altomare D, Hui Y, Fan D. Emodin Bidirectionally Modulates Macrophage Polarization and Epigenetically Regulates Macrophage Memory. J. Biol. Chem. 2016;291(22): 11491-503.

[160] Woods MW, Zahoor MA, Dizzell S, Verschoor CP, Kaushic C. Medroxy-progesterone acetate-treated human, primary endometrial epithelial cells reveal unique gene expression signature linked to innate immunity and HIV-1 susceptibility. Amer. J. Rep. Immunol. 2018;79(1).

[161] Ye J, Xu B, Fan B, Zhang J, Yuan F, Chen Y, et al. Discovery of Selenocysteine as a Potential Nanomedicine Promotes Cartilage Regeneration With Enhanced Immune Response by Text Mining and Biomedical Databases. Front. Pharmacol. 2020;11:1138.

[162] Behjati S, Tarpey PS. What is next generation sequencing? Arch. Disease Childhood Ed. Pract. Ed. 2013;98(6): 236-8.

[163] Dulanto Chiang A, Dekker JP. From the Pipeline to the Bedside: Advances and Challenges in Clinical Metagenomics. J. Infect. Dis. 2020;221(Supplement_3): S331-s40.

[164] Lucan C, Pop LA, Florian A, Pileczki V, Petrushev B, Dima D, et al. HLA Genotyping using Next Generation

Sequencing. Roman. J. Internal Med. 2016;54(2):98-104.

[165] Tomuleasa C, Selicean C, Cismas S, Jurj A, Marian M, Dima D, et al. Minimal residual disease in chronic lymphocytic leukemia: A consensus paper that presents the clinical impact of the presently available laboratory approaches. Crit. Rev. Clin. Lab. Sci. 2018;55(5):329-45.

[166] Woollard PM, Mehta NA, Vamathevan JJ, Van Horn S, Bonde BK, Dow DJ. The application of next-generation sequencing technologies to drug discovery and development. Drug Discov. Today. 2011;16(11-12):512-9.

[167] Braicu C, Buiga R, Cojocneanu R, Buse M, Raduly L, Pop LA, et al. Connecting the dots between different networks: miRNAs associated with bladder cancer risk and progression. J. Exp. Clin. Cancer Res. 2019;38(1):433.

[168] Ciocan-Cârtiță CA, Jurj A, Raduly L, Cojocneanu R, Moldovan A, Pileczki V, et al. New perspectives in triple-negative breast cancer therapy based on treatments with TGFβ1 siRNA and doxorubicin. Mol. Cell. Biochem. 2020;475(1-2):285-99.

[169] Rubin A, Salzberg AC, Imamura Y, Grivitishvilli A, Tombran-Tink J. Identification of novel targets of diabetic nephropathy and PEDF peptide treatment using RNA-seq. BMC genomics. 2016;17(1):936.

[170] Ng SB, Buckingham KJ, Lee C, Bigham AW, Tabor HK, Dent KM, et al. Exome sequencing identifies the cause of a mendelian disorder. Nat. Genet. 2010;42(1):30-5.

[171] Sas V, Pasca S, Jurj A, Pop L, Muramatsu H, Ono H, et al. MicroRNA-155-5p Plays a Critical Role in Transient Leukemia of Down Syndrome by Targeting Tumor Necrosis Factor Receptor Superfamily Members. Cell. Physiol. Biochem. 2020;54(5):994-1012.

[172] Wang Z, Li Y, Hou B, Pronobis MI, Wang M, Wang Y, et al. An array of 60,000 antibodies for proteome-scale antibody generation and target discovery. Science advances. 2020;6(11):eaax2271.

[173] Petric RC, Pop LA, Jurj A, Raduly L, Dumitrascu D, Dragos N, et al. Next generation sequencing applications for breast cancer research. Clujul Med. 2015;88(3):278-87.

[174] NCCN Clinical Practice Guidelines in Oncology: Non-Small Cell Lung Cancer [Internet]. NCCN. 2020 [cited Accsessed on 17.08.2020]. Available from: https://www.nccn.org/professionals/physician_gls/pdf/nscl.pdf.

[175] NCCN Clinical Practice Guidelines in Oncology. Colon Cancer [Internet]. NCCn. 2020 [cited 17 August 2020]. Available from: https://www.nccn.org/professionals/physician_gls/pdf/colon.pdf.

[176] NCCN Clinical Practice Guidelines in Oncology. Breast and ovarian cancer [Internet]. NCCN. 2020 [cited 17 August 2020]. Available from: https://www.nccn.org/professionals/physician_gls/pdf/genetics_bop.pdf.

[177] Treon SP, Xu L, Guerrera ML, Jimenez C, Hunter ZR, Liu X, et al. Genomic Landscape of Waldenström Macroglobulinemia and Its Impact on Treatment Strategies. J. Clin. Oncol. 2020;38(11):1198-208.

[178] Tshibangu-Kabamba E, Ngoma-Kisoko PJ, Tuan VP, Matsumoto T, Akada J, Kido Y, et al. Next-Generation Sequencing of the Whole Bacterial Genome for Tracking Molecular Insight into the Broad-Spectrum Antimicrobial Resistance of Helicobacter pylori Clinical Isolates from the Democratic Republic of Congo. Microorganisms. 2020;8(6).

[179] Butler DJ, Mozsary C, Meydan C, Danko D, Foox J, Rosiene J, et al. Shotgun Transcriptome and Isothermal Profiling of SARS-CoV-2 Infection Reveals Unique Host Responses, Viral Diversification, and Drug Interactions. bioRxiv. 2020:2020.04.20.048066.

[180] Ureshino H, Koarada S, Kamachi K, Yoshimura M, Yokoo M, Kubota Y, et al. Immune dysregulation syndrome with de novo CTLA4 germline mutation responsive to abatacept therapy. Int. J. Hematol. 2020;111(6):897-902.

[181] Schatz S, Falk M, Jóri B, Ramdani HO, Schmidt S, Willing EM, et al. Integration of Tumor Mutation Burden and PD-L1 Testing in Routine Laboratory Diagnostics in Non-Small Cell Lung Cancer. Cancers. 2020;12(6).

[182] Pop LA, Cojocneanu-Petric RM, Pileczki V, Morar-Bolba G, Irimie A, Lazar V, et al. Genetic alterations in sporadic triple negative breast cancer. Breast. 2018;38:30-8.

[183] Klowak JA, El Helou S, Pernica JM, Parker MJ, Surette M, Poinar H, et al. Fast I(n)dentification of Pathogens in Neonates (FINDPATH-N): protocol for a prospective pilot cohort study of next-generation sequencing for pathogen identification in neonates with suspected sepsis. BMJ Paediat. Open. 2020;4(1):e000651.

[184] McConnell L, Houghton O, Stewart P, Gazdova J, Srivastava S, Kim C, et al. A novel next generation sequencing approach to improve sarcoma diagnosis. Modern Pathol. 2020;33(7):1350-9.

[185] Yang F, Anekpuritanang T, Press RD. Clinical Utility of Next-Generation Sequencing in Acute Myeloid Leukemia. Mol. Diagn. Ther. 2020;24(1):1-13.

[186] Dy GK, Nesline MK, Papanicolau-Sengos A, DePietro P, LeVea CM, Early A, et al. Treatment recommendations to cancer patients in the context of FDA guidance for next generation sequencing. BMC Med. Inform. Decis. Mak. 2019;19(1):14.

[187] Farnaes L, Wilke J, Ryan Loker K, Bradley JS, Cannavino CR, Hong DK, et al. Community-acquired pneumonia in children: cell-free plasma sequencing for diagnosis and management. Microbiol. Infectious Disease. 2019;94(2):188-91.

[188] Farrow E, Rengasamy Venugopalan S, Thiffault I, Saunders C. Examination of rare genetic variants in dental enamel genes: The potential role of next-generation sequencing in primary dental care. Orthodont. Craniofac. Res. 2019;22 Suppl 1:49-55.

[189] Réda M, Richard C, Bertaut A, Niogret J, Collot T, Fumet JD, et al. Implementation and use of whole exome sequencing for metastatic solid cancer. EBioMedicine. 2020;51:102624.

[190] Goodnow RA, Davie CP. Chapter One - DNA-Encoded Library Technology: A Brief Guide to Its Evolution and Impact on Drug Discovery. In: Goodnow RA, editor. Annual Reports in Medicinal Chemistry. 50: Academic Press; 2017. p. 1-15.

[191] Franzini RM, Neri D, Scheuermann J. DNA-encoded chemical libraries: advancing beyond conventional small-molecule libraries. Aco. Chem. Res. 2014;47(4):1247-55.

[192] Goodnow RA, Jr., Dumelin CE, Keefe AD. DNA-encoded chemistry: enabling the deeper sampling of chemical space. Nat. Rev. Drug Discov. 2017;16(2):131-47.

[193] Neri D, Lerner RA. DNA-Encoded Chemical Libraries: A Selection System Based on Endowing Organic Compounds with Amplifiable Information. Annu. Rev. Biochem. 2018;87:479-502.

[194] Salamon H, Klika Škopić M, Jung K, Bugain O, Brunschweiger A. Chemical Biology Probes from Advanced DNA-encoded Libraries. ACS Chem. Biol. 2016;11(2):296-307.

[195] Lemke M, Ravenscroft H, Rueb NJ, Kireev D, Ferraris D, Franzini RM. Integrating DNA-encoded chemical libraries with virtual combinatorial library screening: Optimizing a PARP10 inhibitor. Bioorganic Med. Chem. Lett. 2020;30(19):127464.

[196] Reidenbach AG, Mesleh MF, Casalena D, Vallabh SM, Dahlin JL, Leed AJ, et al. Multimodal small-molecule screening for human prion protein binders. J. Biol. Chem. 2020.

[197] Cuozzo JW, Clark MA, Keefe AD, Kohlmann A, Mulvihill M, Ni H, et al. Novel Autotaxin Inhibitor for the Treatment of Idiopathic Pulmonary Fibrosis: A Clinical Candidate Discovered Using DNA-Encoded Chemistry. J. Med. Chem. 2020;63(14):7840-56.

[198] Dawadi S, Simmons N, Miklossy G, Bohren KM, Faver JC, Ucisik MN, et al. Discovery of potent thrombin inhibitors from a protease-focused DNA-encoded chemical library. Proc. Natl. Acad. Sci. U.S.A. 2020;117(29):16782-9.

[199] Kung PP, Bingham P, Burke BJ, Chen Q, Cheng X, Deng YL, et al. Characterization of Specific N-α-Acetyltransferase 50 (Naa50) Inhibitors Identified Using a DNA Encoded Library. ACS Med. Chem. Lett. 2020;11(6):1175-84.

[200] Arakaki AK, Tian W, Skolnick J. High precision multi-genome scale reannotation of enzyme function by EFICAz. BMC genomics. 2006;7:315.

[201] Verdine GL, Walensky LD. The challenge of drugging undruggable targets in cancer: lessons learned from targeting BCL-2 family members. Clin. Cancer Res. 2007;13(24):7264-70.

[202] Passiglia F, Malapelle U, Del Re M, Righi L, Pagni F, Furlan D, et al. KRAS inhibition in non-small cell lung cancer: Past failures, new findings and upcoming challenges. Eur. J. Cancer. 2020;137:57-68.

[203] Kato S, Okamura R, Sicklick JK, Daniels GA, Hong DS, Goodman A, et al. Prognostic implications of RAS alterations in diverse malignancies and impact of targeted therapies. Int. J. Cancer. 2020;146(12):3450-60.

[204] Duffy MJ, Crown J. Drugging "undruggable" genes for cancer treatment: Are we making progress? Int. J. Cancer. 2020.

[205] Zhou J, Zhao W, Wu J, Lu J, Ding Y, Wu S, et al. Neoantigens Derived from Recurrently Mutated Genes as Potential Immunotherapy Targets for Gastric Cancer. BioMed Res. Int. 2019;2019:8103142.

[206] Duffy DJ, Krstic A, Halasz M, Schwarzl T, Fey D, Iljin K, et al. Integrative omics reveals MYCN as a global suppressor of cellular signalling and enables network-based therapeutic target discovery in neuroblastoma. Oncotarget. 2015;6(41):43182-201.

[207] Ng CK, How KY, Tee KK, Chan KG. Characterization and Transcriptome Studies of Autoinducer Synthase Gene from Multidrug Resistant Acinetobacter baumannii Strain 863. Genes. 2019;10(4).

[208] Subramanian D, Natarajan J. RNA-seq analysis reveals resistome genes and signalling pathway associated with vancomycin-intermediate *Staphylococcus aureus*. Ind. J. Med. Microbiol. 2019;37(2):173-85.

[209] Chou S. Approach to drug-resistant cytomegalovirus in transplant recipients. Curr. Opin. Infect. Dis. 2015;28(4):293-9.

[210] Port JA, Wallace JC, Griffith WC, Faustman EM. Metagenomic profiling of microbial composition and antibiotic

resistance determinants in Puget Sound. PloS one. 2012;7(10):e48000.

[211] Leprohon P, Fernandez-Prada C, Gazanion É, Monte-Neto R, Ouellette M. Drug resistance analysis by next generation sequencing in Leishmania. Int. J. Parasitol. Drugs Drug Resist. 2015;5(1):26-35.

[212] Lee ER, Parkin N, Jennings C, Brumme CJ, Enns E, Casadellà M, et al. Performance comparison of next generation sequencing analysis pipelines for HIV-1 drug resistance testing. Sci. Rep. 2020;10(1):1634.

[213] Fogel JM, Bonsall D, Cummings V, Bowden R, Golubchik T, de Cesare M, et al. Performance of a high-throughput next-generation sequencing method for analysis of HIV drug resistance and viral load. J. Antimicrob. Chemother. 2020.

[214] Sivay MV, Palumbo PJ, Zhang Y, Cummings V, Guo X, Hamilton EL, et al. HIV drug resistance, phylogenetic analysis, and superinfection among men who have sex with men and transgender women in sub-Saharan Africa: HPTN 075. Clinical Infect. Dis. 2020.

[215] Noguera-Julian M, Lee ER, Shafer RW, Kantor R, Ji H. Dry Panels Supporting External Quality Assessment Programs for Next Generation Sequencing-Based HIV Drug Resistance Testing. Viruses. 2020;12(6).

[216] Ávila-Ríos S, Parkin N, Swanstrom R, Paredes R, Shafer R, Ji H, et al. Next-Generation Sequencing for HIV Drug Resistance Testing: Laboratory, Clinical, and Implementation Considerations. Viruses. 2020;12(6).

[217] Patel MC, Mishin VP, De La Cruz JA, Chesnokov A, Nguyen HT, Wilson MM, et al. Detection of baloxavir resistant influenza A viruses using next generation sequencing and pyrosequencing methods. Antiviral research. 2020;182:104906.

[218] Ye L, Meng F, Mao X, Zhang Y, Wang J, Liu Y, et al. Using next-generation sequencing to analyze Helicobacter pylori clones with different levofloxacin resistances from a patient with eradication failure. Medicine. 2020;99(32):e20761.

[219] Cho WC, Shin YK, Na YS, Ryu MH, Ku JL, Kang YK. The role of novel fusion genes in human GIST cell lines derived from imatinib-resistant GIST patients: A therapeutic potential of fusion gene. Biochem. Biophys. Res. Commun. 2020;529(3):699-706.

[220] Wishart DS, Knox C, Guo AC, Shrivastava S, Hassanali M, Stothard P, et al. DrugBank: a comprehensive resource for in silico drug discovery and exploration. Nucleic Acids Res. 2006;34(Database issue):D668-72.

[221] Wishart DS, Knox C, Guo AC, Cheng D, Shrivastava S, Tzur D, et al. DrugBank: a knowledgebase for drugs, drug actions and drug targets. Nucleic Acids Res. 2008;36(Database issue):D901-6.

[222] Wishart DS. Discovering drug targets through the web. Comparative biochemistry and physiology Part D, Genomics & proteomics. 2007;2(1): 9-17.

[223] Chang C, Bahadduri PM, Polli JE, Swaan PW, Ekins S. Rapid identification of P-glycoprotein substrates and inhibitors. Drug Metabol. Disposit. 2006;34(12):1976-84.

[224] Jolivette LJ, Ekins S. Methods for predicting human drug metabolism. Advances in clinical chemistry. 2007;43:131-76.

[225] Li H, Gao Z, Kang L, Zhang H, Yang K, Yu K, et al. TarFisDock: a web server for identifying drug targets with docking approach. Nucleic Acids Res. 2006;34(Web Server issue):W219-24.

[226] Chong CR, Sullivan DJ, Jr. New uses for old drugs. Nature. 2007; 448(7154):645-6.

[227] Jiang T, Kong B, Yan W, Wu C, Jiang M, Xu X, et al. Network Pharmacology to Identify the Pharmacological Mechanisms of a Traditional Chinese Medicine Derived from Trachelospermum jasminoides in Patients with Rheumatoid Arthritis. Med. Sci. Monitor. 2020;26:e922639.

[228] Lokhande KB, Doiphode S, Vyas R, Swamy KV. Molecular docking and simulation studies on SARS-CoV-2 M(pro) reveals Mitoxantrone, Leucovorin, Birinapant, and Dynasore as potent drugs against COVID-19. J. Biomol. Struct. Dynam. 2020:1-12.

[229] Mazzolari A, Gervasoni S, Pedretti A, Fumagalli L, Matucci R, Vistoli G. Repositioning Dequalinium as Potent Muscarinic Allosteric Ligand by Combining Virtual Screening Campaigns and Experimental Binding Assays. Int. J. Mol. Sci. 2020;21(17).

[230] Thomas RE. Optimising Seniors' Metabolism of Medications and Avoiding Adverse Drug Events Using Data on How Metabolism by Their P450 Enzymes Varies with Ancestry and Drug-Drug and Drug-Drug-Gene Interactions. J. Personal. Med. 2020;10(3).

[231] Xu C, Ke Z, Liu C, Wang Z, Liu D, Zhang L, et al. Systemic in Silico Screening in Drug Discovery for Coronavirus Disease (COVID-19) with an Online Interactive Web Server. J. Chem. Inf. Model. 2020.

[232] Ramachandran B, Jeyakanthan J, Lopes BS. Molecular docking, dynamics and free energy analyses of Acinetobacter baumannii OXA class enzymes with carbapenems investigating their hydrolytic mechanisms. J. Med. Microbiol. 2020.

[233] Khelfaoui H, Harkati D, Saleh BA. Molecular docking, molecular dynamics simulations and reactivity, studies on approved drugs library targeting ACE2 and SARS-CoV-2 binding with ACE2. J. Biomol. Struct. Dynam. 2020:1-17.

[234] Wei TZ, Wang H, Wu XQ, Lu Y, Guan SH, Dong FQ, et al. In Silico Screening of Potential Spike Glycoprotein Inhibitors of SARS-CoV-2 with Drug Repurposing Strategy. Chinese J. Integr. Med. 2020:1-7.

[235] Fabbri C, Kasper S, Zohar J, Souery D, Montgomery S, Albani D, et al. Drug repositioning for treatment-resistant depression: Hypotheses from a pharmacogenomic study. Progress Neuro-psychopharmacol. Biol. Psych. 2020;104:110050.

[236] Lu X, Wu X, Jing L, Tao L, Zhang Y, Huang R, et al. Network Pharmacology Analysis and Experiments Validation of the Inhibitory Effect of JianPi Fu Recipe on Colorectal Cancer LoVo Cells Metastasis and Growth. Evidence-based complementary and alternative medicine : eCAM. 2020;2020:4517483.

[237] Li T, Liu Q, Zhang R, Liao Q, Zhao Y. Identification of prognosis-related genes and construction of multi-regulatory networks in pancreatic cancer microenvironment by bioinformatics analysis. Cancer Cell Int. 2020;20:341.

[238] Fiorucci D, Milletti E, Orofino F, Brizzi A, Mugnaini C, Corelli F. Computational drug repurposing for the identification of SARS-CoV-2 main protease inhibitors. J. Biomol. Struct. Dynam. 2020:1-7.

[239] Ibrahim MAA, Abdelrahman AHM, Hegazy MF. In-silico drug repurposing and molecular dynamics puzzled out potential SARS-CoV-2 main protease inhibitors. J. Biomol. Struct. Dynam. 2020:1-12.

[240] Masoudi-Sobhanzadeh Y, Masoudi-Nejad A. Synthetic repurposing of drugs against hypertension: a datamining method based on association rules and a novel discrete algorithm. BMC Bioinform. 2020;21(1):313.

[241] Huang B, Xiong J, Zhao X, Zheng Y, Zhu N. Network Pharmacology-Based Analysis of the Pharmacological Mechanisms of Aloperine on Cardiovascular Disease. Evidence-based complementary and alternative medicine : eCAM. 2020;2020:5180716.

[242] Zhao Z, Li J, Li H, Yuan Wu NY, Ou-Yang P, Liu S, et al. Integrative Bioinformatics Approaches to Screen Potential Prognostic Immune-Related Genes and Drugs in the Cervical Cancer Microenvironment. Front. Genet. 2020;11:727.

[243] Chandra A, Gurjar V, Ahmed MZ, Alqahtani AS, Qamar I, Singh N. Exploring potential inhibitor of SARS-CoV2 replicase from FDA approved drugs using insilico drug discovery methods. J. Biomol. Struct. Dynam. 2021:1-8.

[244] Gupta Y, Maciorowski D, Zak SE, Jones KA, Kathayat RS, Azizi SA, et al. Bisindolylmaleimide IX: A novel anti-SARS-CoV2 agent targeting viral main protease 3CLpro demonstrated by virtual screening pipeline and in-vitro validation assays. Methods (San Diego, Calif). 2021.

[245] Kwarteng A, Asiedu E, Sakyi SA, Asiedu SO. Targeting the SARS-CoV2 nucleocapsid protein for potential therapeutics using immuno-informatics and structure-based drug discovery techniques. Biomed. Pharmacother. 2020;132:110914.

[246] Mok PL, Koh AE, Farhana A, Alsrhani A, Alam MK, Suresh Kumar S. Computational drug screening against the SARS-CoV-2 Saudi Arabia isolates through a multiple-sequence alignment approach. Saudi J. Biol. Sci. 2021.

[247] Anwar F, Altayb HN, Al-Abbasi FA, Kumar V, Kamal MA. The computational intervention of macrolide antibiotics in the treatment of COVID-19. Curr. Pharmaceut. Design. 2021.

[248] Fiscon G, Conte F, Farina L, Paci P. SAveRUNNER: A network-based algorithm for drug repurposing and its application to COVID-19. PLoS computational biology. 2021;17(2): e1008686.

[249] Song L, Xiao G, Tang R, Zhang X, Gao Z, Sun S, et al. Next-generation sequencing and RT-PCR to identify a 32-day SARS-CoV-2 carrier. Clinical chemistry and laboratory medicine. 2021.

[250] Papoutsis A, Borody T, Dolai S, Daniels J, Steinberg S, Barrows B, et al. Detection of SARS-CoV-2 from patient fecal samples by whole genome sequencing. Gut pathogens. 2021;13(1):7.

[251] Armero A, Berthet N, Avarre JC. Intra-Host Diversity of SARS-Cov-2 Should Not Be Neglected: Case of the State of Victoria, Australia. Viruses. 2021;13(1).

[252] Charre C, Ginevra C, Sabatier M, Regue H, Destras G, Brun S, et al. Evaluation of NGS-based approaches for SARS-CoV-2 whole genome characterisation. Virus Evol. 2020;6(2):veaa075.

[253] Panzera Y, Ramos N, Frabasile S, Calleros L, Marandino A, Tomás G, et al. A deletion in SARS-CoV-2 ORF7 identified in COVID-19 outbreak in Uruguay. Transbound. Emerg. Dis. 2021.

[254] Tushir S, Kamanna S, Nath SS, Bhat A, Rose S, Aithal AR, et al. Proteo-Genomic Analysis of SARS-CoV-2: A Clinical Landscape of Single-Nucleotide Polymorphisms, COVID-19 Proteome, and Host Responses. J. Proteome Res. 2021.

[255] Gunadi, Wibawa H, Marcellus, Hakim MS, Daniwijaya EW, Rizki LP, et al. Full-length genome characterization and phylogenetic analysis of SARS-CoV-2 virus strains from Yogyakarta and Central Java, Indonesia. PeerJ. 2020;8:e10575.

[256] Wei J, Alfajaro MM, DeWeirdt PC, Hanna RE, Lu-Culligan WJ, Cai WL, et al. Genome-wide CRISPR Screens Reveal Host Factors Critical for SARS-CoV-2 Infection. Cell. 2021;184(1):76-91.e13.

Section 2

Rational Drug Design

Chapter 5

The Rational Drug Design to Treat Cancers

Abdul Hameed Khan

Abstract

Professor Ross of London University, England, was using nitrogen mustard to treat cancers by attacking both strands of tumor DNA. As a part of my doctoral thesis, I am to design drugs using aziridine to attack only one strand of DNA. Over the years, I made over 100 dinitrophenyl aziridine derivatives. One of them is dinitrobenzamide (CB1954) which gives a CI of 70, highest toxicity to animal tumor ever recorded. CB1954 wipes out a solid aggressive tumor by attacking a single-strand DNA of Walker carcinoma 256, in rat. My greatest challenge at NCI in USA is to translate the animal work which I did in London University to humans. As radiolabeled methylated quinone crosses the blood-brain barrier in mice, I decided to use quinone moiety as a carrier for aziridine rings to attack glioblastomas, the brain tumor in humans. By attaching two aziridines and two carbamate moieties to quinone, I made AZQ (US Patent 4,146,622). By treating brain cancer with AZQ, we observed that glioblastoma tumor not only stops growing but also starts shrinking. Literature search showed that AZQ is extensively studied.

Keywords: drug design, tumor treatment, novel drugs for cancer treatment

1. Introduction

Rational drug design is absolutely essential for developing novel drugs for treating any disease, especially cancers. Our Institute, the NIH (National Institutes of Health is an agency of US Government) learned this fact by spending enormous amount of money over the years by testing known and unknown products obtained by synthesis or from plants and animals on a variety of testing tumor systems. The discovery of a handful of drugs by trial and errors at a cost of millions was considered a waste of time and money. In early days, we absorbed the losses because our Institute, located about 10 miles from Washington, DC, is the largest biomedical center in the world. Our annual budget is over 40 billion dollars per year. Over 26 institutes have about 3000 labs where about 21,000 scientists work in 50 buildings. My lab was in the National Cancer Institute (NCI), which is the largest among all institutes and it has a budget of over 5 billion dollars per year. Now, we became more cautious screening drugs. About 20% of our budget is spent in-house and the 80% of our budget is provided to research labs around the world by reviewing their research projects by expert panels called the study sections to approve funds to projects most rational and most likely to be accomplished.

2. Genomic medicine

This chapter describes the novel drug design based on the genetic makeup of a patient. My main focus is on two major areas, and they are diagnostic and novel drug design to treat these diseases. Today, we are treated with the same medicine for the same disease as if we all have the identical genomes. In fact, no two people look alike and no two genomes are alike. Our genome is made of six billion four hundred million nucleotides, and in almost every 1000 nucleotides, we find a variant and in the entire script, we find 3.4 million variants called the SNP (single-nucleotide polymorphism). Each of us has a unique genetic makeup and requires the development of a specific medicine to treat that disease. This concept is now known as the pharmacogenomic, and it provides a paradigm shift in drug design.

To design a genomic medicine, first we need to sequence the whole genome identifying specific region (genes) which codes for specific proteins. Second, we need to sequence as many genomes as possible (such efforts are undergoing as a Thousand Genome Project, a Million or a Three Million Genome Project) to compare their sequences to identify differences called variants. Then, we need to develop next generation of sequencers to sequence everyone's genome as cheaper and as faster as possible. Next, we need to identify the differences in the genetic scripts, and then, we need to separate bad or abnormal mutated variants responsible for causing diseases. Next, we need to identify rare variants as diagnostic tools responsible for causing rare diseases (young people diseases) such as Parkinson, Huntington, cystic fibrosis, muscular dystrophy, color blindness, sickle cell anemia, etc. called the monogenic or Mendelian diseases. Next, we need to identify the common genetic diseases (old people diseases) such as cancers, cardiovascular diseases, and Alzheimer. First, we generate sequence data and then by comparing we find a correlation between variants and diseases. We can construct a correlation map of all variants responsible for causing all genetic disorders. After diagnosing the diseases, the next most important step is to treat those diseases by novel drug design.

Our work below describes over a quarter of a century's effort by first designing drugs to shut off genes responsible for causing cancers in animals and then we further describe how we translated the animal work in humans. The following pages describe the development of genomic medicine based on the drug design and on the genetic makeup of a patient. I will cover three areas. First, I will provide historical background which describes the early development of medicines to treat diseases. Second, I will describe the rational drug design to treat abnormal mutated genes and the specific nucleotide identified by the human genome sequencing to develop new drugs to treat old diseases, and finally, I will discuss the ethical problems in an attempt to answer the consequences of prolonging human life on planetary resources and environment.

3. Historical background

Since the dawn of human civilization, achieving human longevity has been the dream of every King, every Queen, every Pharos, and every Caesar. But they all died in their 50s by infectious diseases. Then came the science and technology revolution. In 1928, Alexander Flaming, while working on influenza virus, observed that a mold had developed accidently on a staphylococcus culture plate. By killing the bacteria, the mold had created a bacteria-free circle around itself. He was so inspired by the presence of the bacterial free zone that he conducted further experiment and found that the mold culture produced a substance which prevented growth of staphylococci, even when diluted 800 times. He named the active substance penicillin. The discovery of penicillin [1] was followed by a host of new antibiotics such as streptomycin, neomycin, kanamycin, paromomycin, apramycin, tobramycin, amikacin, netilmicin, and gentamicin and dozens of their derivatives which wipeout Gram-positive and Gram-negative bacteria. Misuse and overuse of antibiotics in agriculture resulted in the bacterial resistance. For example, farmers overuse the antibiotics in food-producing animals not only to kill the bacteria in cows, goat, and chicken farms but also use to promote growth in these animals exposing excessive amount of antibiotics residues to humans in their food. We developed a spectroscopic method [2] to detect their residue in PPT (parts per trillion) to provide safe food for consumption.

We conquered infectious diseases. We increased our life span from 50 to 60 years. Then came the genetic revolution. We broke the genetic code and unlocked the secrets of life. Now, we are ready to manipulate life not only to clean up our environmental pollution but also to produce new food, new fuel, and new medicine to treat every disease known to mankind. We also succeeded in increasing human lifespan beyond 60 to 70 years.

Next, we read the entire book of human life. We read the total genetic information that makes the human life; we completed the Human Genome Project. Next, we sequenced the human genome, that is, we read the number of nucleotides and the order in which they are arranged. With advancement in science and technology, we sequenced the human genome cheaper and faster using the next-generation sequencers such as nanopore. Then, we completed the 1000 Human Genome Project. We are able to compare the reference sequence of every gene with the 1000 copies of the same gene from different individuals to identify differences. These differences are called variants. If the good variant came from the pancreas, it produces insulin which is used to treat diabetes. If the variant came from an abnormal mutated gene, it is responsible for causing common diseases such as cancers, cardiovascular diseases, or Alzheimer. Soon, we will prepare a variant map of the entire genome to identify all 6000 diseases; then, we can design drugs to treat these diseases by shutting off their genes. The Thousand Genome Project will help us single out the rare mutation responsible for causing rare genetic diseases such as Parkinson with precision and accuracy. With advent of new technologies, we embark on the more ambitious project such as The Human Brain Project and The Human Longevity Project.

Next, I will attempt to answer an important question about how to design drugs to treat diseases to save human life by using the information available from the Human Genome Project. How many diseases we inherit from our parents? We identified good and bad genes in our genome. We wonder if bad mutations are written on our DNA. Is the secret hidden in the long string of four nucleotides text on a three-letter codon carrying 24,000 genes in 46 chromosomes in our genome containing six billion four hundred million nucleotides? Could we identify the genetic variants responsible for our diseases by comparing the whole-genome sequence of the centenarians with the 1000 Human Genome Project completed by US and a Million Human Genome Project to be completed by European and a three Million Human Genome Project announced by the Chinese to identify rare alleles responsible for causing rare diseases with accuracy and precision. We want to identify in the whole genome the specific genetic variations and the few nucleotides responsible for our health. As I said above, before the discovery of antibiotics, most people died in their 50s. Today, all infectious diseases are treated with antibiotics. Now, we must treat the old age common diseases such as cancers, cardiac diseases, and Alzheimer. To save human life from these dreadful diseases, we have to design drugs to shut off genes responsible for causing these old age diseases. Next, I will describe how I design drugs to shut off genes which cause brain cancer, glioblastomas. Similar rationale could be used to design drugs to shut off genes responsible for causing cardiovascular diseases and Alzheimer.

4. Genotype-phenotype correlations

Our genes are units of inheritance and carry instructions to make proteins, and when the proteins fold, they become reactive and carry out a specific function. Hundreds of proteins interact to make a cell, and millions of cells interact to make a tissue. Hundreds of tissues interact to make an organ, and several organs interact to make a human being. We carry in our body 220 different tissues. The instructions to make tissues are written in our genes. A defected tissue could be identified by looking at the mutation in the genes. We can prevent diseases at a very early stage of our lives. By sequencing a fertilized egg, the genotype, we could identify the mutations responsible for future diseases in tissues, the phenotype. If a patient has a family history of a specific disease, to prevent future generation from inheriting the disease, it is best advice for such families to have conception by in vitro fertilization after making sure that the fertilized egg is free from all abnormal mutations responsible for causing the disease.

Our entire genome, the book of our life, is written in four nucleotides, and they are A (adenine), T (thiamine), G (guanine), and C (cytosine). The chain of these nucleotides forms a double-stranded string of nucleotides, one strand is inherited from our mother and another from our father, running in opposite directions called the DNA (deoxyribonucleotide). According to Francis Crick's Central Dogma [3], double-stranded DNA is transcribed into a single-stranded RNA which is translated in the ribosome into proteins. The discovery of the double helical structure of DNA explained how the information to create life is stored, replicate, evolved, and passed on to the next generation. This discovery opened a new world order of ideas and buried the old explanation of the magical mystical appearance of life on Earth.

The double-stranded DNA explained that the essence of life is information and the information is located on these four nucleotides. Every set of three nucleotides on the mRNA forms a codon which codes for a specific amino acid. The four-letter text of nucleotides forms a three-letter codon which codes for an amino acid. There are 64 different combinations of codons which codes for all 20 amino acids. Sequencing human genome identifies the number of nucleotides and the order in which they are arranged. Less than 2% of our genome contains regulatory region, a piece of DNA, which controls the function of genes. More than 300 regulatory regions have been identified. More than 98% of our genome contains non-coding region used to be called the junk DNA which makes up to 60% of our entire genome. The non-coding regions contains repetitive piece of DNA, which is tightly packed and mostly remain silent. The sequencing of this region showed that the non-coding region is the part of viruses and bacteria picked up by our genome during the millions of years of our evolutionary process. During bacterial or viral infection, the non-coding DNA could unfold transcribing into RNA resulting into hazardous protein which could create havoc for our health.

Genes are the unit of inheritance. As I said above, out of four-letter text, that is A-T and G-C, and three letters code for an amino acid called the codon. The starting codon in a gene is the codon AUG (instead of T nucleotide, we use U nucleotide because thiamin is converted to more water-soluble uracil), which codes for amino acid methionine. Long chain of DNA synthesis begins. The starting codon is followed by a series of hundreds of codons which codes for different amino acids in different species. There are three stop codons, and they are AUG, UGG, and UGA.

Once the stop codons appear, DNA synthesis stops. Bacteria and viruses have short codon chain. The longest chain is in a gene of Duchenne muscular dystrophy, a neurological disease whose chain extends to two and a half million codons. Once a gene is identified, using restriction enzymes, like EcoR1, we can cut, paste, and copy all genes individually making a restriction site map. Once a single gene is isolated, we could compare the sequence of this gene with the Thousand Genome Project to identify abnormal mutation responsible for the disease and design drugs to shut off that gene. Sequencing is like extracting gold from its ore.

Let us examine the sequence of the genome of human egg and sperm. An egg contains a single strand of 164 million nucleotide bases carrying 1144 genes, while the human sperm contains a single strand of 59 million nucleotide bases carrying 214 genes. When comparing the sequence of an egg or sperm with sequence of the 1000 eggs and sperms of different people, we notice changes. These changes are called variants. These variants are mutations caused by radiations, chemical and environmental pollution, viral infection, or genetic inheritance resulting in rare diseases. Once a bad gene is identified, sequencing will identify the abnormal nucleotide. Now, we can design drug to bind to this nucleotide and shut off its function. We present in the "Cancers" section below a novel drug design. Using aziridines and carbamate how we design drugs to shut off these genes to restore health.

Although we are allowed to shut off and remove bad genes, we are not allowed to introduce good genes in the egg and sperm to enhance the abilities of egg and sperm because modification introduced in the egg and sperm will pass on to the next 1000 generations. For this reason, germ line gene therapy is forbidden in all countries. At this time, we cannot answer a simple question. Are we to determine the quality of life of individuals who will not even be born before the century is over?

We cannot design novel drugs unless we find the abnormal mutations responsible for causing that disease. The reading of the total genetic information that makes us human is called the human genome. The reading of the entire book of our life is authorized by the US Congress under The Human Genome Project. It will answer the most fundamental question we have asked ourselves since the dawn of human civilization. What does it mean to be human? What is the nature of memory and our consciousness? Our development from a single cell to a complete human being? The biochemical nature of our senses and the process of our aging? The scientific basis of our similarity and dissimilarity: similarity is that all living creatures from a tiny blade of grass to the mighty elephant including man, mouse, monkey, mosquitos, and microbes are all made of the same chemical building blocks, yet we are so diverse that no two individuals are alike even identical twins are not exactly identical, they grow up to become two separate individuals.

In 1990, US Congress authorized 3 billion dollars to NIH to decipher the entire human genome under the title, "The Human Genome Project." We found that our genome contains six billion four hundred million nucleotide bases, half comes from our father and another half comes from our mother. Less than 2% of our genome contains genes which code for proteins. The other 98% of our genome contains switches, promoters, terminators, etc. The 46 chromosomes present in each cell of our body are the greatest library of the Human Book of Life on planet Earth. The chromosomes carry genes which are written in nucleotides. Before sequencing (determining the number and the order of the four nucleotides on a chromosome), it is essential to know how many genes are present on each chromosome in our genome. The Human Genome Project has identified not only the number of nucleotides on each chromosome but also the number of genes on each chromosome [4–8].

The following list provides the details composition of each chromosome including the number of nucleotides and the number of genes on each chromosome.

We found that chromosome-1 is the largest chromosome carrying 263 million A, T, G, and C nucleotide bases and has only 2610 genes. Chromosome-2 contains 255 million nucleotide bases and has only 1748 genes. Chromosome-3 contains 214 million nucleotide bases and carries 1381 genes. Chromosome-4 contains 203 million nucleotide bases and carries 1024 genes. Chromosome-5 contains 194 million nucleotide bases and carries 1190 genes. Chromosome-6 contains 183 million nucleotide bases and carries 1394 genes. Chromosome-7 contains 171 million nucleotide bases and carries 1378 genes. Chromosome-8 contains 155 million nucleotide bases and carries 927 genes. Chromosome-9 contains 145 million nucleotide bases and carries 1076 genes. Chromosome-10 contains 144 million nucleotide bases and carries 983 genes. Chromosome-11 contains 144 million nucleotide bases and carries 1692 genes. Chromosome-12 contains 143 million nucleotide bases and carries 1268 genes. Chromosome-13 contains 114 million nucleotide bases and carries 496 genes. Chromosome-14 contains 109 million nucleotide bases and carries 1173 genes. Chromosome-15 contains 106 million nucleotide bases and carries 906 genes. Chromosome-16 contains 98 million nucleotide bases and carries 1032 genes. Chromosome-17 contains 92 million nucleotide bases and carries 1394 genes. Chromosome-18 contains 85 million nucleotide bases and carries 400 genes. Chromosome-19 contains 67 million nucleotide bases and carries 1592 genes. Chromosome-20 contains 72 million nucleotide bases and carries 710 genes. Chromosome-21 contains 50 million nucleotide bases and carries 337 genes. Chromosome-22 contains 56 million nucleotides and carries 701 genes. Finally, the sex chromosome of all female called the (X) contains 164 million nucleotide bases and carries 1141 genes. The male sperm chromosome contains 59 million nucleotide bases and carries 255 genes.

If you add up all genes in the 23 pairs of chromosomes, they come up to 26,808 genes and yet we keep on mentioning 24,000 genes needed to keep us function normally. As I said above, a gene codes for a protein, not all 24,000 genes code for proteins. It is estimated that less than 19,000 genes code for protein. Because of the alternative splicing, each gene codes for more than one protein. All functional genes in our body make less than 50,000 proteins which interact in millions of different ways to give a single cell. Millions of cells interact to give a tissue, hundreds of tissues interact to give an organ, and several organs interact to make a human.

Not all genes act simultaneously to make us function normally. Current studies show that a minimum of 2000 genes are enough to keep human function normally; the remaining genes are backup support system and they are used when needed. The non-functional genes are called the pseudo genes. For example, millions of years ago, humans and dogs shared some of the same ancestral genes; we both carry the same olfactory genes, only in dogs, they still function to search for food. Since humans do not use these genes to smell for searching food, these genes are broken and lost their functions, but we still carry them. We call them pseudo genes. Recently, some Japanese scientists have activated the pseudo genes; this work may create ethical problem in future as more and more pseudo genes are activated. Nature has good reasons to shut off those pseudo genes.

Next, we converted the analog language biology to the digital language of computer, that is, from A-T and G-C nucleotides to numbers 0 and 1. Now, we can write a program and design a computer to read the book of life faster and faster. Today, we can read our entire genome in 1 day at a cost of 1000 dollars. We can also upload our digitized genome on the computer. Once uploaded on the Website, our genome could travel with the speed of light to anywhere in the world or in the universe.

Once the good and bad genes are identified, we learned that the good genes code for good proteins which keep us healthy and the bad genes produce bad proteins that make us sick. Using good genes, we make good protein to treat diseases such as insulin is used to treat diabetes. On the other hand, we could identify bad gene and design drugs to shut off bad genes to prevent diseases. This starts a new era of genomic medicine based on differences of the genetic make of each individual.

The double-stranded DNA in the normal cell, the autosome, is retained with the individual. When the person dies, the genome dies with him. On the other hand, the DNA in a germ line cell lives on for generations. Through egg and sperm cells, the DNA is passed on to the future generations, that is, the information is passed on from parents to the fetus in different combinations for generation after generation.

A sperm, the Y-chromosome, is made of a single string of 59 million nucleotide bases and carry 231 genes, while an egg, the X-chromosome, is made of a single string of 164 million nucleotide bases and carry 1144 genes. Neither two sperms nor any two eggs are alike. Once the egg is fertilized, the nucleotides and genes are exchanged (recombination occurs) among nucleotides forming a double-stranded DNA. Now, each string is a complete genome. During replication, each string separates and picks up the complimentary nucleotide bases (such as nucleotide A picks up T and G picks up C) from the nucleotide pool and forms two double-stranded DNA forming two daughter cells. The two strands of each chain run in opposite directions.

5. Reactive and predictive medicine

Reactive medicine is the treatment of a disease after its symptoms are revealed and the full-blown disease appears. During your annual health checkup, your physicians order a number of tests. For example, if you are a 40-year-old male and go to the doctor, he prescribed a PSA (prostate-specific antigen) test for the early signs of prostate cancer, if you are a 40-year-old woman, your doctor prescribes the mammograms for the early signs of breast cancer, and if you are 50 years old, he prescribes the colonoscopy for colon cancer. Once the symptoms are revealed, the standard treatment is prescribed for a disease such as surgery, radiations treatment, or chemotherapy. The treatment after the appearance of its symptoms is considered as the reactive medicine.

A specific example is as follows: suppose your physician finds that you are sick with high temperature and high blood pressure, he prescribes Plavix a medicine of standard treatment for lowing your blood pressure and temperature. It is a reactive medicine. You receive treatment after your illness is diagnosed. Plavix is a useful drug for treating high blood pressure, but it does not respond in 15% of the patients. In treating reactive medicine, we do not really know what is going on in the body of those patients until after sequencing their genome, and identifying the abnormal mutation in their genetic makeup and then designing drugs to treat those patients is the true genomic medicine.

Predictive medicine, on the other hand, is the treatment of a disease long before its onset by examining your normal genomic script of the effected organ from your book of life and comparing its entire script with the genome of a sick patient. Spelling errors in our genome are the mutations responsible for causing diseases. The difference between the reactive medicine and the predictive medicine is whether you have the disease or you will come down with the disease because you are carrying a mutation which could become activated and make you sick. Genomic medicine will have predictive quality. When comparing genome sequences, we find differences called variants. Good variants are responsible for our evolution, and abnormal variants are responsible for causing diseases. Using restriction enzymes (molecular scissors) like EcoR1, we can cut, paste, and copy a gene (conduct genetic engineering) and prepare a chart (called restriction site map) of all 6000 variants responsible for causing all 6000 diseases. By comparing the sequence of a genes from the chart, we can predict which specific gene variant is expected to cause which disease.

As cells grow, the mutations accumulate and defects in genotype manifests in phenotype. By using MRI (magnetic resonance imaging which provides three-dimensional image) method, one could see the progressive microscopic abnormal changes in the nucleotide bases and predict the onset of a disease. The three-dimensional MR imaging could serve as a diagnostic technique. Once the diagnosis is confirmed, drug design must begin to treat the disease. There are 220 different tissues in our body. We take the MRI of all 220 tissues of a healthy person and during his annual medical checkup compare the present MRI with the previous years' MRI to see any unusual microscopic changes predicting diseases. Once identified, the next logical step is to design drugs to shut off mutated genes to prevent diseases.

Genetic disorders can be caused by a mutation in one gene (monogenic disorder), by mutations in multiple genes (multifactorial inheritance disorder), by a combination of gene mutations and environmental factors, or by damage to chromosomes (changes in the number of copies or structure of entire chromosomes, or part of the chromosome that carries genes). What specific nucleotide damage forming the codon is responsible for causing catastrophic diseases? By comparing the mutations in a DNA sequence (genotype), we can predict the onset of a disease in human (phenotype). The microscopic changes not detected by observations can be confirmed by three-dimensional MRI technique, which will diagnose diseases long before the symptoms appear.

To some degree, we have achieved the quantity control of the population by genome sequencing. Western countries are far ahead of the Eastern nations. The sequencing of the human genome provides rational approach to the quality control of the population. We have good news for those families who are suffering from severe heritable diseases generations after generations. Some of those rare allele diseases are mental diseases such as Parkinson, Huntington, schizophrenia, bipolar disorder, etc. often known as the Mendelian diseases. Those family members can still have children, but we recommend that they have conception by in vitro fertilization, that is, they conceived children outside their bodies, that is, in the test tube. The fertilized egg is harvested in the incubators for 3 days until it grows from a single cell to eight number cells. Without any ill effect, one cell could be removed and its genome is sequenced. Suppose the sequenced cell identify abnormal mutations when implanted will produce an incurably blind child or mentally retarded child. Is there a reason to bring this child into this intensely competitive world? Education is a very long process. To complete his education from age 5 to 25 years, when he completes his education and receives his Doctorate Degree, a child has to take several tests. If he fails one test, he is thrown out of the success train. No matter how painful it is on either religious or moral ground, we must ask ourselves a simple question. Does this fertilized ovum produce an acceptable member of the human society? If the answer is no, then we must throw out the defected ovum and use a new ovum. Out of eight, we have screened only a single cell. Should we sequence and select a cell for implantation which is free from all harmful mutations? Will society approve this reasonable request?

5.1 Drug design for rare allele diseases

These are the diseases of people of all ages. Before the development of antibiotics, most people died of infectious diseases around age 50. First, antibiotics, penicillin (discovered by Alexander Fleming), was used for treating wounds before the WWII. As I said above, enormous funds were made available by the army to develop large-scale antibiotics to treat wounded soldiers returning from the battle ground during WWII. During the following decades, novel class of aminoglycoside antibiotics were discovered, which are valuable therapeutic agents. Some of them are streptomycin, neomycin, kanamycin, paromomycin, apramycin, tobramycin, amikacin, netilmicin, gentamicin, etc. Dozens of their water/fat-soluble derivatives were synthesized. They are considered broad spectrum antibiotics because they inhibit the growth of both Gram-negative and Gram-positive bacteria causing deadly diseases and save human life. All aminoglycoside antibiotics are relatively small, basic, and water-soluble molecules that form stable salts. Most aminoglycoside antibiotics are products of fermentation of filamentous actinomycetes of the genus *Streptomyces*.

5.2 Drug design for common allele diseases

These are the diseases of old age people. Nowadays, people rarely die of infectious diseases. Because of the availability of a variety of antibiotics, today, most people live beyond age 70 years and some of them go on living beyond 80 years of age. Those who live beyond 70 are faced with three major old age diseases, which are responsible for causing the death of most patients during their lifetime and they are cancers, cardiac diseases, and Alzheimer. These are genetic diseases and could be treated either by gene therapy (using CRISPER technology by replacing bad gene with the good gene using CRISPER-Cas9) or by drug therapy. There are about 3000 monogenic diseases and could be treated by replacing the defected gene with good gene, that is, by gene therapy or designing drugs to shut off the bad genes that is drug therapy. Gene therapy cannot be applied to treat multiple genetic defects such as Alzheimer, cancer, and cardiovascular diseases. Drug therapy could be used to develop novel treatments. Recently completed 1000 Human Genome Project identify with precision and accuracy the genes responsible for causing these diseases. It is now possible to design drugs to shut off these genes and save human life. Genes code for proteins and a mutated gene codes for abnormal proteins resulting in these diseases.

6. Cancers

Cancer is the leading cause of death and has surpassed the death of cardiovascular diseases. Over 636,000 people died of cancer; 1.9 million new cases will be diagnosed this year including 78,000 prostate cancer, 40,000 breast cancer, 16,000 lung and bronchus cancer, and 15,000 colon and rectal cancer. Once diagnosed by gene sequencing, the next step is to design drug to shut off those genes.

6.1 The rational drug design to treat cancers

All three old age diseases, that is, cancer, cardiovascular diseases, and Alzheimer carry multiple mutated genes responsible for causing these diseases. In each of the above three diseases, it is the mutated genes that code for wrong protein which causes these diseases. If we design drugs to shut off mutated genes in one disease, using the same rationale, we should be able to shut off bad genes in all three old age diseases. Although coronary artery disease is a complex disease, researchers have found about 60 genomic variants that are present more frequently in people with coronary artery disease. Most of these variants are dispersed across the genome and do not cluster on one specific chromosome. Drugs are designed to seek out the specific malignant gene, which replicates faster producing acids. Aziridines and carbamate moieties are sensitive to acid. Drugs carrying the aziridines and carbamate moieties are broken down in acidic media generating carbonium ions which attack DNA shutting off genes. Only the acid producing genes will be attacked no matter where they are located. It does not matter whether they are clustered or dispersed across genome.

The supreme intellect for drug design is Ross, an Englishman, who is a Professor of Chemistry at the London University. Professor WCJ Ross is also the Head of Chemistry Department at the Royal Cancer Hospital, a postgraduate medical center of the London University. Ross was the first person who designed drugs for treating cancers. He designed drugs to cross-link both strands of DNA that we inherit one strand from each parent. Cross-linking agents such as nitrogen mustard are extremely toxic and were used as chemical weapon during the First World War. More toxic derivatives were developed during the Second World War. Using the data for the toxic effect of nitrogen mustard used during the First World War, Ross observed that soldiers exposed to nitrogen mustard showed a sharp decline of white blood cells (WBC) that is from 5000 cell/CC to 500 cells/CC. Children suffering from childhood leukemia have a very high WBC count over 90,000 cells/CC. In sick children, most of the WBCs are premature, defected, and unable to defend the body from microbial infections. Ross rationale was that cancer cells divide faster than the normal cell, by using nitrogen mustard to cross-link both strands of DNA, one can control and stop the abnormal WBC cell division in leukemia patients. It was indeed found to be true. Professor Ross was the first person to synthesize a large number of derivatives of nitrogen mustard. By using an analog of nitrogen mustard, called chlorambucil [9], he was successful in treating childhood leukemia. In America, two physicians named Goodman and Gilman from the Yale University were the first to use nitrogen mustard to treat cancer in humans. Nitrogen mustards and its analogs are highly toxic. Ross was a chemist; over the years, he synthesized several hundred derivatives of nitrogen mustard molecules to modify toxicity of nitrogen mustard [10–14].

Although analogs of nitrogen mustard are highly toxic, they are more toxic to cancer cells and more cancer cells are destroyed than the normal cells. Toxicity is measured as the chemotherapeutic index (CI), which is a ratio between toxicity to cancer cells versus the toxicity to normal cells. Higher CI means that the drugs are more toxic to cancer cell. Most cross-linking nitrogen mustard have a CI of 10, that is, they are 10 times more toxic to cancer cells. Some of the nitrogen mustard analogs Ross made over the years are useful for treating cancers such as chlorambucil for treating childhood leukemia (which brought down the WBC level down to 5000/CC). Childhood leukemia is the name of a disease occurs in children only. Chlorambucil made Ross one of the leaders of the scientific world. He also made melphalan and myrophine for treating pharyngeal carcinomas [15].

6.2 The discovery of AZQ (US Patent 4,146,622) for treating brain cancer

At the London University, I was trained as an organic chemist in the Laboratory of Professor WCJ Ross of the Royal Cancer Hospital, a postgraduate medical center of the London University. After working for about 10 years at the London University,

I moved to America when I was honored by the Fogarty International Fellowship Award by the National Institutes of Health, NIH, and the National Cancer Institute, NCI, of the USA. NIH has been my home for over a quarter of a century; I designed drugs to shut off mutated genes. All three common allele diseases have genetic origin. The rationale I used to synthesize anticancer drugs could be used to treat the other two old age diseases like Alzheimer and cardiovascular diseases. In the following sections, I will describe in detail how anticancer drug like AZQ was designed to shut off glioblastoma genes which cause brain cancer in humans. Using the same rational, we will consider how each of the other two diseases, namely, cardiovascular disease and Alzheimer could be treated by shutting off their genes to save human life: The order of these diseases are arranged based on the level of funding provided by NIH specifically by the NCI (National Cancer Institute).

As I said above, Professor Ross was designing drugs to attack both strands of DNA simultaneously by cross-linking using nitrogen mustard analogs, which are extremely toxic. As a part of my doctoral thesis, I was assigned a different path. Instead of cross-linking DNA, I am to design drugs to attack only one strand of DNA. This class of drugs is called aziridines. Over the years, I made over 100 dinitrophenyl aziridine derivatives. One of them is dinitrobenzamide (CB1954) which gives a CI of 70, highest ever recorded. CB1954 wipes out a solid tumor by attacking the DNA of Walker carcinoma 256, a solid aggressive tumor in rat.

Nitrogen mustards are highly toxic because they have neither specificity nor selectivity. They attack all dividing cells whether they are normal or abnormal. On the other hand, the analogs of aziridines and carbamates remain inactive in the basic and neutral media. They become activated only in the presence of acidic media.

I used a simple rationale, the aziridine attacks DNA in acidic medium, particularly the N-7 guanine. The dye dinitrobenzamide has great affinity for Walker tumor [16–18]. The aziridine dinitrobenzamide (CB1954) stains the tumor. As the tumor grows, it uses glucose as a source of energy. Glucose is broken down to pyruvic acid. It is the acid which attacks the aziridine ring. The ring opens to generate a carbonium ion, which attacks the most negatively charged N-7 guanine of DNA shutting off the Walker carcinoma gene in rat. To continue my work, I was honored with the Institute of Cancer Research Post-Doctoral Fellowship Award of the Royal Cancer Hospital of London University. To increase the toxicity of CB1954 to Walker carcinoma, I made additional 20 analogs as a postdoctoral fellow. When I attached one more carbonium generating moiety, the carbamate moiety to the aziridine dinitrobenzene, the compound aziridine dinitrobenzamide carbamate was so toxic that its therapeutic index could not be measured. We stopped the work at the London University for the safety concern.

I continued my work on the highly toxic aziridine/carbamate combination in America when I was offered the Fogarty International Fellowship Award to continue my work at the National Cancer Institute (NCI) of the National Institutes of Health (NIH). I brought the idea from London University of attacking one strand of DNA using not only aziridine, but also carbamate without using the same dye dinitrobenzamide [19–21].

My greatest challenge at NCI is to translate the animal work which I did in London University to humans. One day, I came across a paper which described that radiolabeled methylated quinone cross the blood-brain barrier in mice. When injected in mice, the X-ray photograph showed that the entire radioactivity was concentrated in the mice's brain within 24 hours. I immediately realized that glioblastoma multiforme, the brain tumor in humans, is a solid aggressive tumor like Walker carcinoma in rats. I decided to use quinone moiety as a carrier for aziridine rings to attack glioblastomas. By introducing an additional carbamate moiety, I could increase its toxicity several folds. I planned to use this rational to translate animal work to human by introducing multiple aziridine and carbamate moieties to the quinone to test against glioblastomas in humans. Attaching two aziridines and two carbamate moieties to quinone, I made AZQ. By treating brain cancer with AZQ, we observed that glioblastoma tumor not only stop growing but also start shrinking. I could take care of at least one form of deadliest old age cancers, that is, glioblastomas. Literature search showed that AZQ is extensively studied.

As I said above, glioblastoma, the brain cancers, is a solid and aggressive tumor and is caused by mutations on several chromosomal DNA. Mutations on DNA are the result of damaging DNA nucleotides by exposure to radiations, chemical and environmental pollution, viral infections, or genetic inheritance. The other factors responsible for causing DNA mutations are due to the fast rate of replication of DNA. For example, the bacteria *E. coli* grows so rapidly that within 24 hours, a single cell on a petri dish forms an entire colony of millions when incubated on the agar gel. Rapid replication is responsible for introducing genetic defects causing diseases.

When an additional piece of nucleotide is attached to a DNA string, it is called insertion or a piece of DNA is removed from the DNA string; it is called deletion or structural inversion of DNA is responsible for mutations. Since the gene in a DNA codes for proteins, insertion and deletion on DNA have catastrophic effects on protein synthesis. Glioblastomas represent such an example. In glioblastomas, three major changes occur on chromosomes (C-7, C-9, and C-10) and two minor changes occur on chromosomes (C-1 and C-19). These mutations are responsible for causing brain cancers in humans. In a normal human cell, chromosome-7 which is made of 171 million nucleotide base pairs and carries 1378 genes. When insertion occurs on chromosome-7, 97% of glioblastoma patients are affected by this mutation. On the other hand, a different mutation occurs on chromosome-9 which is made of 145 million nucleotide base pairs and it carries 1076 genes. A major deletion of a piece of DNA occurs on chromosome-9, which results in 83% patients who are affected by this mutation. A minor deletion of DNA also occurs on chromosome-10 which is made of 144 million base pairs and it carries 923 genes. Although it is a minor deletion of a piece of DNA, it contributes to 91% patients with glioblastoma. To a lesser extent, small mutation occurs on chromosome-1 (the largest chromosome in our genome). It is made of 263 million nucleotide base pairs and carries 2610 genes), and chromosome-19 (it is made of 67 million base pairs and carries 1592 genes) is also implicated in some forms of glioblastomas.

All known glioblastomas causing genes are located on five different chromosomes and carries a total of 9579 genes. It appears impossible to design drugs to treat glioblastomas since we do not know which nucleotide on which gene and on which chromosome is responsible for causing the disease. With the completion of 1000 Human Genome Project, it becomes easier. By simply comparing the patient's chromosomes with the 1000 genomes, letter by letter, word by word, and sentence by sentence, we could identify the difference called the variants with precision and accuracy, the exact variants or mutations responsible for causing the disease. Once the diagnosis is confirmed, the next step is how to treat the disease.

With the quinone ring, I could introduce different combinations of aziridine rings and carbamate moieties and could create havoc for glioblastomas. My major concern was how toxic this compound would be to the human brain cells. Fortunately, brain cells do not divide, only cancer cells divide.

Our rational drug design work began in the University of London, England, and completed in the Laboratory of the National Cancer Institute (NCI), of the National Institutes of Health (NIH), in Bethesda, Maryland, USA. Over this period, we conducted over 500 experiments which resulted in 200 novel drugs. They were all tested against the experimental animal tumors. Forty-five of them were considered valuable enough to be patented by the US Government (US Patent 4,146,622). One of them is AZQ. Radiolabeled studies showed that AZQ has the ability to cross organ after organ, cross the blood-brain barrier, cross the nuclear membrane, and attack the nuclear DNA shutting off the gene. X-ray studies showed that the radioactivity is concentrated in the tumor region. Glioblastoma stop growing and start shrinking. For the discovery of AZQ, I was honored with the "2004 NIH Scientific Achievement Award," one of America's highest awards in Medicine and I was also honored with the India's National Medal of Honor, "Vaidya Ratna," a gold medal (see **Figures 1–4**).

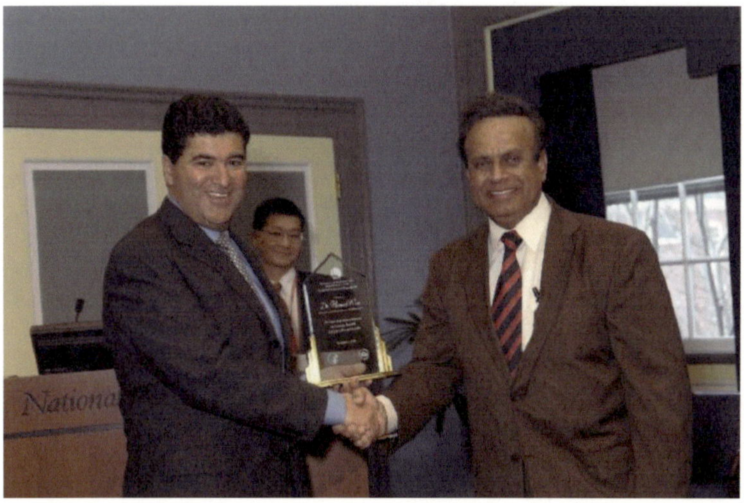

Figure 1.
2004 NIH Scientific Achievement Award presented to Dr. Hameed Khan by Dr. Elias Zerhouni, the director of NIH during the NIH/APAO award ceremony held on December 3, 2004. Dr. Khan is the discoverer of AZQ (US Patent 4,146,622), a novel experimental drug specifically designed to shut off a gene that causes brain cancer for which he receives a 17-year royalty for his invention (license number L-0I9-0I/0). To this date, more than 300 research papers have been published on AZQ. The award ceremony was broadcast live worldwide by the Voice of America (VOA). Dr. Khan is the first Indian to receive one of America's highest awards in Medicine.

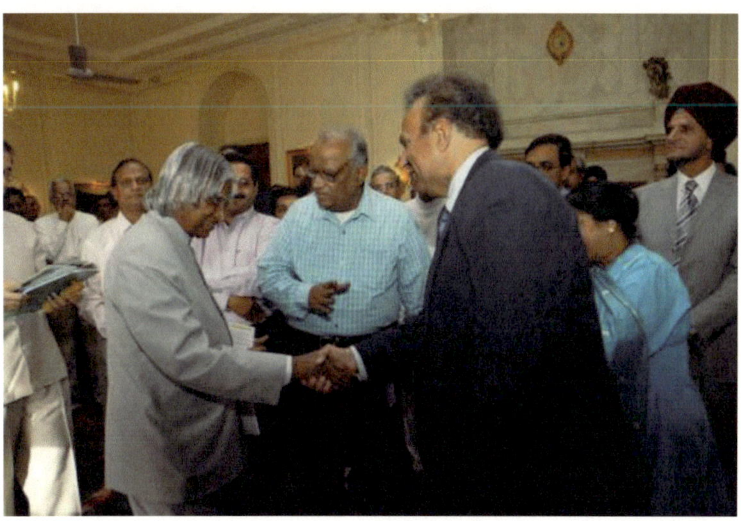

Figure 2.
His excellency, Dr. A.P.J. Abdul Kalam, the President of India greeting Dr. A. Hameed Khan, discoverer of anticancer AZQ, after receiving 2004, Vaidya Ratna, the gold medal, one of India's highest awards in Medicine at the Rashtrapati Bhavan (Presidential Palace), in Delhi, India, during a reception held on 02 April 2004.

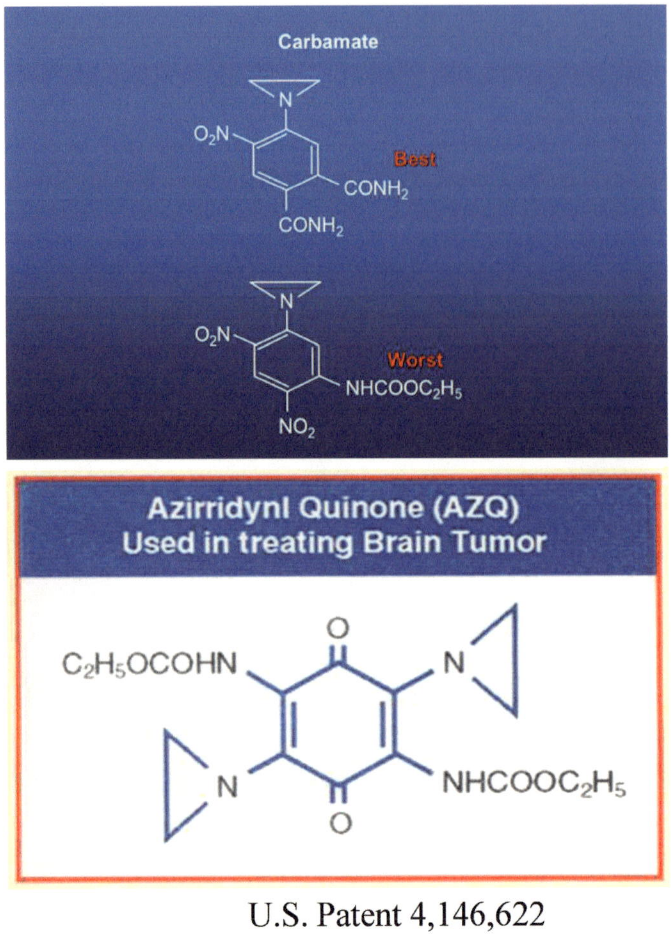

Figure 3.
Single-strand DNA binding aziridine and carbamate.

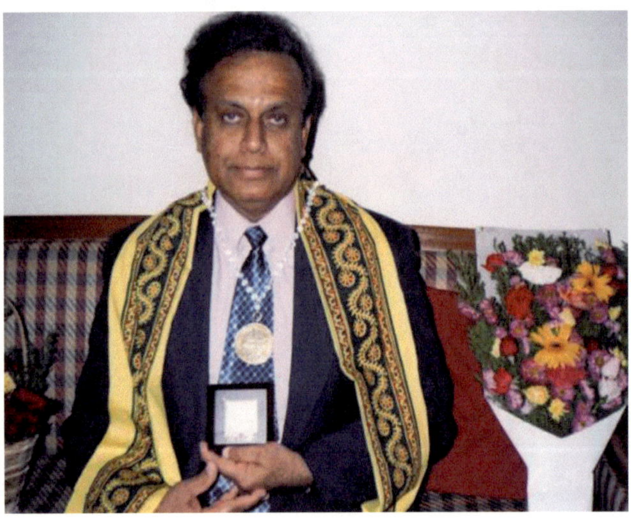

Figure 4.
Gold medal for Dr. Khan. Dr. A. Hameed Khan, a scientist at the National Institutes of Health (NIH), USA, an American scientist of Indian origin was awarded on April 2, 2004. Vaidya Ratna, the gold medal, one of India's highest awards in Medicine for his discovery of AZQ (US Patent 4,146,622) which is now undergoing clinical trials for treating bran cancer.

7. Cardiovascular diseases

Coronary artery disease is complex involving about 60 genomic variants (genes). All variants are not clustered on any specific chromosome. These variants are dispersed across the entire genome. Although all variants have not been sequenced, we can shut off only the mutated gene without knowing the sequence of all other genes. As I mentioned above in the "Cancers" section, the mutated gene grows rapidly forming the tumor. As it grows, it uses glucose as a source of energy, which is broken down to produce pyruvic acid. In the presence of acid, the analogs of aziridine and carbamate are activated to generate carbonium ion which attack the tumor DNA shutting off their genes. While we may someday be able to sequence all 60 genes associated with the coronary artery disease, presently, we can single out and identify the mutated gene bound complex using radiolabeled aziridine and carbamate. The following example explains how some arrhythmias causing genes could be identified and how drug could be designed to shut off these genes.

The term "QT" refers to the segment of an electrocardiogram, which measures the duration of time for the heart to relax after a heartbeat. In long QT syndrome, the duration of time is abnormally prolonged and creates a vulnerability to dangerous arrhythmias [22]. Ever since the syndrome was described in 1957, researchers have engaged in a genetic race to identify the genes associated with long QT syndrome, which currently includes 17 genes. Three genes, *KCNQ1*, *KCNH2*, and *SCN5A*, had sufficient evidence to be implicated as "definitive" genetic causes for typical long QT syndrome. Four other genes had strong or definitive evidence supporting their role in causing atypical forms of long QT syndrome, presenting in the newborn symptoms associated with heart block, seizures, or delays in development. Once the mutated genes are identified, we could design drugs to shut off these genes as described in the "Cancers" section.

8. Alzheimer

In 1906, the German physician scientist Dr. Alois Alzheimer identified the microscopic changes in the brain of a patient with the memory loss. He was the first physician to identify the disease in a 50-year-old woman who suffered from psychosis and who died within 4 years. Using special dyes, he stained the brain tissues which carried abnormal protein deposit around her brain which controlled brain function. He identified two kinds of legions of amyloid patches which he mistakenly thought was fatty patches and now turned out to be proteins. He observed a patch of fatty deposit on the top of the brain cells called plaques and the legions inside the nerve cells called tangles. He accurately correlated the abnormal protein deposits around brain cells with the controlled of brain function [23–26].

Today, we know that the age is the single most risk factor for developing Alzheimer. By age 65 or older, the risk for developing Alzheimer is about 10%, and by age 85 or older, the risk factor is as high as 40 or 50%. As people grow old, they become senile. When he performed the autopsy of many senile persons, Dr. Alzheimer found the same plaques and tangles in many other samples. Early onset or late onset of Alzheimer resulted in the epidemic of Alzheimer. When comparing a normal brain with the Alzheimer brain, we find that the Alzheimer brain has shrunken and there is a concentration of plaques and tangles in neurons. In healthy brain cells, we see occasional plaques and tangles. It defines the disease; the plaque and tangles start building up as we grow old, and over years and decades, the symptoms begin to develop. Symptoms include memory loss and decrease in ability of learning and recall. Early onset affects cognition which encompasses memory and other mental functions such as erosion of attention, thinking, reasoning, visual functions, spatial function, and dementia with memory loss and other cognitive functions resulting in mental impairment which affects to the degree interfering with the daily life.

Recent studies confirm that Alzheimer is an irreversible brain disorder which slowly destroys memory and thinking skills. The damage to the brain is not particularly associated to any specific gene, but the presence of the one form of the apolipoprotein E (APOE) is a suspect gene whose presence does increase a patient's risk for developing Alzheimer. The early onset of Alzheimer is associated with three single gene mutations: first, the presence of an amyloid precursor protein (APP) located on chromosome-21; the presence of presenilin 1 (PSEN1) on chromosome-14 and the presence of presenilin 2 (PSEN2) located on chromosome-1. All three chromosomes are very large and carry hundreds of genes. For example, chromosome-1 is the largest chromosome in the genome. It is made of 163 million nucleotide bases carrying 2610 genes. Chromosome-21 is made of 50 million nucleotide bases carrying 337 genes, while chromosome-14 is made of 109 million nucleotide bases carrying 1173 genes.

A recent 7 million Utah population study identified two additional genes RAB10 located on chromosome-2 (which is made of 155 million nucleotide bases and carry 1798 genes) and SAR1A gene located on chromosome-10 (which is made of 144 million nucleotide bases and carry 983 genes) associated with the formation of plaques and tangles. Mutations on these genes may be associated with the onset of Alzheimer.

Of all the genes on these chromosomes, only five single-gene mutations are associated with the early onset of the Alzheimer, it is the greatest challenge to design drugs to attack only the mutated genes. As I said above in the "Cancers" section, the good news is that the only mutated genes grow rapidly using glucose as a source of energy. Glucose is broken down to produce pyruvic acid. It is the acid which activates the aziridine and carbamate moieties producing powerful carbonium ion which attack N-7 guanine of DNA and shut off only the mutated genes. Other genes are not affected. Using C-14 radiolabeled aziridines, we can identify the mutated gene which form the aziridine/protein complex as described in the "Cancers" section.

9. Rationale for designing drugs to treat Alzheimer

It is well known that using the TFT dye, which is 3,6-dimethyl-2-(4-dimethlaminophenyl)-benzothiazoline, could be used to stain the plaques and tangles of Alzheimer tissues. Using TFT dye as a carrier for the aziridine and carbamate moieties, we could design drugs to attack the mutated DNA to shut off genes which form plaques and tangles to prevent the progress of Alzheimer.

In the above "Cancers" section, I have described in detail how I had used quinone as a carrier for aziridine and carbamate ions in designing AZQ to attack the brain tumor DNA to shut off genes for treating brain cancer. Similarly, the analogs of benzothiazoline dyes could be used to carry aziridine and carbamate moieties to attack the plaque and tangle DNA and shut off genes responsible for causing Alzheimer.

10. What other cancers should we explore next?

Could I use the same rational drug design and introduce a novel method for treating breast tumor?

Although mutations on BRCA1 gene located on chromosome-17 (which is made of 92 million nucleotide bases carrying 1394 genes) have been identified years ago responsible for causing breast cancer, we wonder why it has been so difficult to design drugs on rational basis to treat breast cancer. By the time the breast cancer diagnosis is confirmed in a patient, the BRCA1 has accumulated more than 3000 mutations. Genotyping of the blood would also show the existence of many cells carrying mutated cells responsible for creating secondary deposits. It is also believed that by the time breast cancer is confirmed, metastatic cancer cells have already been spread from liver lung on its way to brain. Since all other organs including breast and liver could be removed and replaced by organ transplant except brain, I thought that protecting brain is utmost important to save life. Once AZQ is developed to protect the brain, I could focus on the breast and prostate cancers.

Recent, radiolabeled studies showed that male hormone testosterone has great affinity for female organs like breast, ovary, and fallopian tube cells. On the other hand, estrogen, the female hormone, has great affinity for male prostate gland. By attaching multiple aziridine rings and carbamate ions to both hormones, I could design novel drugs to attack the breast and the prostate cancer. Now, I found that I could go even further by attaching more than four aziridine and carbamate moieties to both male and female hormones.

In a breast tumor, within the start and stop codons, BRCA1 gene has captured over 200,000 nucleotide bases. The BRCA1 genes carry about 3000 mutations. These mutations are caused by exposure to radiations, chemical or environmental pollutants, viral infection, or genetic inheritance. To attack the mutated nucleotides among the 3000 cells in BRCA1 gene, I could use male hormone, testosterone, and bind multiple radiolabeled aziridine and carbamate ions to attack BRCA1 mutations. By using three-dimensional MRI, I could show how many radiolabeled nucleotides were bound to which mutations. Out of 17 positions available for substitutions on testosterone ring system, there are only three positions, that is, 1, 3, and 17 available for substitution on testosterone ring system. Carl Djerassi [27] had demonstrated that we could activate positions 9 and 10 by reacting with bromoacetamide which introduces a bromo ion on position 10 which could be de-brominated by collidine to introduce a 9,10 double bond which we could further brominate to produce 9,10 dibromo compound. This bromo ion could be replaced by additional aziridine or carbamate ions. I could increase or decrease the number of aziridine and carbamate ions to get the maximum benefit by further brominating positions 15 and 16 to introduce additional aziridine and carbamate moieties.

Similarly, I could use the female hormone estrogen and by attaching multiple aziridine and carbamate ions to attack prostate tumor. Since there are 17 positions also available on estrogen ring as well; again, I could increase or decrease the number of aziridine and carbamate ions to get the maximum benefit.

11. Ethical issues (the impact of science on society)

By 2050, novel drug design would have produced new class of medicine to treat all known 6000 genes. We would not only produce new treatment but also we would have new food, new fuel, and new medicine to treat every disease known to mankind to protect, preserve, and prolong human life beyond 100 years. This section discusses the impact of prolonging human life beyond 100 years.

Our attempt to prolong human life by shutting off the genes of the old age diseases raises several ethical and moral questions. We face the same population problem when we succeed in shutting off genes of all three old age diseases, that is, cancer, cardiovascular disease, and Alzheimer. Most people will live longer and happier life. It raises several questions. What happens after we achieve that goal of reaching 100 years? What would be the quality of our life? By exercises and good nutrition, if the body mass is not retained, the centenarians are most likely to be fragile and weak. They need the help of caretakers to perform the daily routine. By 2050, if we increase the age of about 100 years of about a billion people, we need another billion caretakers. Will the society be happy with this achievement? I doubt it. The society is hardly likely to accept such a proposal.

To cure diseases to prolong human life, several present and future attempts are described below.

We need to make two rationale approaches: first, to identify rare allele in the genome of centenarians responsible for prolonging their lives. Once identified the allele, we need to conduct genetic engineering, that is, to cut, paste, copy, and splice the allele into the genome of volunteers to study its function. Second approach is to design drugs to shut off genes of old age to prolong life.

Next attempt to increase human life would be to prevent the loss of telomeres, the six-letter code (TTAGGG) that shorten our DNA and shorten our lifespan. During replication, each chromosome loses about 30 telomeres each year. If we prevent the loss of telomeres by using the enzyme telomerase reverse transcriptase (TRT), we could slow down the aging process. We have already demonstrated in the worm *C. elegance* that we could increase its lifespan several fold. Now, we could translate this work in human being; we could try by making a less virulent flu virus carrying TRT gene when injected to a volunteer who comes down with a mild flu. When he recovers from the flu, the TRT gene would have inserted in the entire genome of every cell in his body (we can confirm the insertion by sequencing). Suppose at each replication, only 15 telomeres are deleted instead of 30 telomeres. This person is likely to live twice as long. Also, suppose the sequencing of his genome would confirm that every cell of his body carries the TRT gene. Since the longevity treatment with the flu virus is safe, inexpensive, and would be easily available to everyone, should we provide the treatment to every man, woman, and child on the face of the Earth?

Such studies are likely to raise two serious ethical questions. First, we have to ask ourselves, do people have a right to live and second do we have a right to live as long as we wish, no matter how old, how weak, or how sick we are? The answer to first question is, according to the UN charter, we all have the right to life, liberty, and pursuit of happiness. It is the second question which is troublesome. Do people have a right to extent their lives as long as they wish? Most people are reluctant to answer this question either No or Yes. Both answers have some support.

Those who said No have a good reason. First, they argue that there are seven and a half billion people live on planet Earth and we are adding 90 million additional people each year. According to UN estimate, by 2050, the population of the world is likely to reach 9 billion. Does our planet Earth have all resources to support such a population explosion? Can we provide food, fuel, and medicine to all the people of the world? In poor countries, millions are starving now. By extending life, we will have serious problems such as lawlessness, riots, and chaos in the streets. The current population of Earth has polluted the water, the air, and the land. Today, they wonder if the water they drink is safe, the food they eat is safe, and the air they breathe is safe. If we continue to pollute the planet with the current rate which is 110 million ton of pollutant that we release in the atmosphere each year, how much pollutants we would accumulate in the atmosphere in 10 years or in 100 years.

On the other hand, those who say Yes; we should extend life have good reasons as well. We have no Plan B to save human life on some other planet. We look up to Heaven to find another home for humanity. To search for a suitable planet for human life to survive, we need to train an army of astronauts to travel into deep space with extended life span. They may have to travel for centuries to find a habitable planet for humans. We do not want them to die on their way to find a new home for humanity. We must continue to search for treatment to prolong human life.

What if we succeed tomorrow in developing treatment of all three old age diseases to double or triple our lifespan? If we do not succeed tomorrow may be day after tomorrow. Say the treatment is safe, inexpensive, and easily available to every man, woman, and child on the face of the Earth. Who decide that person A will receive the longevity treatment and will live and person B will not receive the same treatment and therefore will die? We need debate and discussion and come up with guidelines for our society. One person cannot provide answer to all these questions. All I want to do is to raise these questions in your mind. My aim will be fulfilled if I have made you think along these lines.

Author details

Abdul Hameed Khan
NCMRR (National Center for Medical Rehabilitation Research), National Institutes of Health (NIH), Bethesda, Maryland, USA

*Address all correspondence to: hameedkhan111@comcast.net

References

[1] Penicillin: The medicine with the greatest impact on therapeutic outcomes. Applied Microbiology and Biotechnology;**92**(4):677-687

[2] Khan AH, Shaikh B, Allen EH, Sokoloski EA. Californium-252 plasma desorption mass spectrometry of aminoglycoside antibiotics. Biomedical and Environmental Mass Spectrometry. 1988;**17**:329-335

[3] Watson JD, Crick FHC. A structure for deoxyribose nucleic acid. Nature. 1953;**171**:737-738

[4] Nature. 2001;**409**:934-941

[5] Nature. 2001;**409**:660-921

[6] Nature. 2004;**431**:931-945

[7] Nature. 2005;**438**:803-810

[8] Nature. 2017;**550**:345-353

[9] Chlorambucil. Cancer Connect News. [Accessed: 21 December 2015]

[10] Ross W.C.J, "The chemistry of cytotoxic alkylating agents" In Advances in Cancer Research by Greenstein, J.P., and Haddow, A., Academic Press, Inc., New York, , 397-449, (1953)

[11] Ross WCJ. Biological Alkylating Agents. London: Butterworth; 1962

[12] Ross WCJ. Journal of the Chemical Society. 1949;**183**

[13] Ross WCJ. Journal of the Chemical Society. 1950;**2257**

[14] Ross WCJ, Mitchley BCV. Annual Report of the British Empire Cancer Campaign. Vol. 421964. p. 70

[15] Lancet;**370**(9594):1209-1218

[16] Cobb LM, Connors TA, Elson LA, Khan AH, Mitchley BCV, Ross WCJ, et al. 2,4-Dinitro-5-ethyleneimino-benzamide (CB 1954): A potent and selective inhibitor of the growth of the Walker carcinoma 256. Biochemical Pharmacology. 1969;**18**:1519-1527

[17] Khan AH, Ross WCJ. Tumor-growth inhibitory nitrophenyl aziridines and related compounds: Structure-activity relationships. Part I. Chemico-Biological Interactions. 1969/70;**1**:27-47

[18] Khan AH, Ross WCJ. Tumour-growth inhibitory nitrophenyl aziridines and related compounds: Structure-activity relationships. Part II. Chemico-Biological Interactions. 1971/72;**4**:11-22

[19] Khan AH, Driscoll JS. Active antitumor components in a decomposed amino sugar. Part 1. Effect of sugar structure on activity. Journal of Pharmaceutical Sciences. 1975;**64**(2):295-299

[20] Hameed Khan A, Driscoll J. Potential central nervous system antitumor agents: Aziridinyl benzoquinones. Part I. Journal of Medicinal Chemistry. 1976;**19**(2):313-317

[21] Chou E, Khan AH, Driscoll J. Potential central nervous system antitumor agents: Aziridinyl benzoquinones. Part II. Aziridinyl quinone: Anti-transplanted tumor agents. Journal of Medicinal Chemistry. 1976;**19**:1302

[22] Clinical Genetics. 2003;**63**(4): 273-282

[23] Arnon R et al. Biochimica et Biophysica Acta. 1991;**1085**(3):336-342

[24] Ji ZS et al. The Journal of Biological Chemistry. 1997;**272**(50):31285-31292

[25] Marcel YL et al. Biochimica et Biophysica Acta. 1983;**750**(2):411-417

[26] Proceedings of the National Academy of Sciences of the United States of America. 2017;**114**(3):E416-E425. DOI: 10.1073/pnas.1612383114

[27] Djerassi C et al. Journal of the American Chemical Society. 1950;**72**:4534

Chapter 6

Natural Medicinal Compounds from Marine Fungi towards Drug Discovery: A Review

Parthiban Brindha Devi and Ridhanya Jayaseelan

Abstract

Marine fungi are species of fungi which live in estuaries environment and marine environment. These species are found in common habitat. Marine fungi are rich in antimicrobial compounds such as anthrones, cephalosporins, peptides, steroids. These compounds which are derived mainly focused in the area of anti-inflammatory, anti-oxidant, anti-fungal, anti-microbial, anti-fouling activity. Bioactive terpene compounds are produced by marine fungi and marine derived fungi can produce sclerotides, trichoderins. Marine fungi have become the richest sources of biologically active metabolites and structurally novel in the marine environment. In a recent study the marine derived fungi *dichotomomyces cejpii* exhibits activity towards cannabinoid which is used to treat alzheimer dementia. *Aspergillus unguis* showed significant acetyl cholinesterase besides its anti-oxidant activity. These acts as a promising intent for discovery of pharmaceutically important metabolites like alkaloids, peptides. Computational (in silico) strategies have been developed and broadly applied to pharmacology advancement and testing. This review summarizes the bioactive compounds derived from marine fungi in accordance with the sources and their biological activities.

Keywords: marine fungi, bioactive compounds, docking, metabolites

1. Introduction

To date there are about 100,000 fungal species, it is expected about one million species that are to be present. In spite of the fact that assessments for the quantity of fungi around 1.5 to more than 5 million, likely less than 10% of fungi have been identified till date. Marine derived fungi are rich in new metabolites [1, 2]. Marine derived fungi consists of secondary metabolites which acts a promising pharmacological and biological properties [3]. Fungi are significant parasites of nutrient cyclers and primary producers. These are tremendously understudied in the marine domain and information on their function is obliged by the fungal dispersion and drivers on worldwide scales [4]. Marine fungi are significant source of secondary metabolites. Despite the fact that marine parasites are less investigated in contrast, various valuable hits have been acquired from the drug discovery point of view adding to their significance in the product discovery [5, 6]. Source of drugs isolated from fungi are being used as camptothecin, torreyanic corrosive, vincristine and cytarabine and paclitaxel. Drug resistance towards diseases like tuberculosis, cancer and HIV-AIDS have been biological target with restricted accomplishment [7]. A few classes of particular metabolites from marine fungi have a wide scope of bio activities against various activities. From marine fungi, more than thousand metabolites have been accounted which can be possibly developed as drugs [8–10]. The source of these marine fungi metabolites is differed as their natural surroundings have been accounted from different sources, for example, algae, sponge, fungi and mangrove derived fungi from bottom residue [11]. Fungi can also be harnessed as sources of chemicals, food and biofuels when people exploit metabolism of fungi [12]. Secondary metabolites are produced by fungi for different purposes, including threat of different pathogens, iron chelation and microorganisms. These metabolites have been recognized from EDF [13]. Isolation of fungi from marine samples has regularly led to the recuperation of microorganisms, which are morphologically, trophically and ecologically like fungi yet are false organisms [14]. Fungi are generally conveyed in marine conditions from intense ocean to polar ice covers. They are found in a wide range of dead and living organic matter. Fungi have been made with those related with sediments, with explicit substrates like algae, driftwood, corals and specifically with sponges [15]. Reliably, fungi confined from sponges represent the biggest number (28%) of novel compounds revealed from marine fungi [16]. In spite of the fact that bio activities of secondary metabolites from marine fungi unveil clinical targets; they are not well constituted for pipelines of drugs and none of them right now is available [17]. To date, in excess of 180 bioactive secondary metabolites got from deep ocean fungi have been reported. These natural metabolites obtained are generally organic and compounds like Pencillium, Polyketides is largely discovered. These incorporate compounds with antimicrobial, anticancer, antiprotozoal, antifungal and antiviral activities [18]. Indeed, even in deep aqueous biological systems, an unsuspected high assorted variety of fungal species was discovered utilizing molecular approaches . At first samples are collected from the ocean. The next step is fungal cultures and sample preparation. In the lab, sterility was acquired by vertical laminar flow hood and bunsen burner. Cultures were allowed to grow aerobically at 25°C with atmospheric pressure and ambient temperature. GYPS medium is used for the growth of strains (1 g glucose, 1 g peptone, 1 g starch 1 g yeast and 30 g ocean salts). Then it is freeze-dried at 80°C. DNA is extracted by homogenizing each sample with sterile glass dabs at 30 rpm. DNA was removed from developed strains with a Fast DNA Spin pack. In Cloning and sequencing, the SSU rRNA qualities were amplified utilizing PCR (primers). Transfer DNA was amplified by PCR at 94°C for 1.30 minutes including 37 cycles of 94°C for 30 s, followed by 48°C for 1.25 min, and 72°C for 1.5 min. The PCR amplification with a last extension step and performed at 72°C for 10 min. The fragments were refined with a High Pure PCR kit (Roche) furthermore, were cloned in the DH5 equipped cells and pGEM-T vector. The two strands was determined utilizing Sequencher 4.6 (GeneCodes), A different grouping arrangement was developed for every phylum utilizing Clustal X 1.81 containing all the databases. After this protocol, 1733 sequences from Basidiomycota,, 4117 sequences from Ascomycota, 215 sequences from Chytridiomycota, 621 sequences from Glomeromycota and 292 sequences from Zygomycota is obtained from various branches of phylogenetic fungal species. Every phylum was then exposed to a numerous grouping arrangement methodology, trailed by neighbor-joining method. Phylogenetic trees were envisioned by utilizing Treeview. The phylogenetic neighbors nearest to the ecological sequence were chosen, and afterward phylogenetic analysis were performed. A different sequence arrangement methodology was performed utilizing CLUSTALX 1.81, and the arrangement was refined by eye. After these evaluation, phylotypes were indicated utilizing a cutoff of 98% (pairwise distance). Then qPCR analysis were performed with 10-μl blends utilizing iQ SYBR green Supermix (Bio-Rad), which contained SYBR green PCR buffer, 2.7 μM dATP, 2.7 μM dGTP, 2.7 μM dCTP,2.7 μM dTTP, and 0.42 U of iTaq DNA polymerase (Bio-Rad). At that point 0.35 μM preliminary MH2 (5′TTCGATGGTAGGATAG3′) and 0.35 μM primer FungqPCR1 (5′TGTCGGGATTGGGTAATTT3′) were added to the blend. Reactions were carried out in optical tubes and were fixed with microseal film. All reactions performed with Chromo 4 thermocycler, utilizing an underlying denaturation at 94°C for 3 min to initiate the compound, trailed by 35 or 40 cycles of denaturation at 94°C for 30 s and furthermore expansion at 48°C for 45 s and afterward by plate perusing. The dissociation curve for temperatures from 65–95°C was estimated after the last qPCR cycle. All informations analyzed utilizing Opticon Monitor 3. Samples which showed the most grounded signals in two starter runs were compared at in a last run. Different plasmid concentrations were utilized to build a standard curve for supreme quantification. Using this formula, standards are found: molecules/μl = a/(plasmid length × 660) × (6.022 × 10^23) where a is the plasmid of concentration in (μg/μl), 6.022 × 10^23 -molar constant, 660- avaerage molecular weight of one base pair [19]. The greater part of the work on secondary metabolites of marine organisms has concentrated on genera, mainly *Penicillium, Aspergillus* and additionally Fusarium and Cladosporium, moreover the less contemplated species merit extraordinary consideration [20]. Biological activity can also be identified using In Silico methods. It gives fast predictions for a large set of compounds in a high-throughput mode. The aim of target discovery is the validation and identification of suitable drug targets for therapeutic intervention and discovery of novel chemical molecules that acts on the most relevant targets for a disease under study. In silico methods include quantitative structure–activity relationships, databases, similarity searching, homology models, pharmacophores, and other molecular modeling, data mining, machine learning, data analysis and network analysis tools that use a computer. Such methods have seen frequent use in the discovery and optimization of physicochemical characterization [21, 22].

2. Secondary metabolites and bioactive compounds

Two new metabolites, *carbonarones* A (1) and B (2), were acquired from the marine-fungi *Aspergillus carbonarius* detached from the marine residue gathered at Weizhou island of China. It indicated moderate cytotoxicity against K562 cells with IC50 estimations of 56.0 and 27.8 μg/ml, individually [23]. 14-norpseurotin A, 29-nordammarane triterpenoid 6β show noteworthy antimicrobial activity against *Bacillus subtilis*, *Escherichia coli* and *Micrococcus lysoleikticus* with MICs of 3.74, 14.97 μM [24]. From the fungi extracts *Ascochyta heteromorpha*, the agent of a foliar infection of oleander (*Nertum oleander*), another cytochalasin named ascochalasin was separated together with deoxaphomin and cytochalasins A and B. Cytochalasins are an enormous gathering of contagious metabolites created by a few genera of fungi which demonstrated diverse biological activities. These compound binds to actin filaments and block the polymerization and also involved in the elongation of actin [25–28]. Three new metabolites, microsphaeropsones A–C (1–3) with an interesting oxepino[2,3-b]chromen-6-one, were detached from the endophytic growth *Microsphaeropsis species* [29] (**Figure 1**).

A semisynthetic dihydrooxepino[2,3-b]chromen6-one 7 was set up by oxidation of the allylic alcohol 1 with manganese dioxide [29]. Marine-derived fungi *Aspergillus versicolor MF160003* for the pharmacologically dynamic secondary metabolites prompts the disclosure of another Xanthenone derivative, 3-hydroxy pinselin, with five known compounds, pinselin,methyl 8-hydroxy-6-methyl-9-oxo-9H-xanthene-1-carboxylate, 2-methoxy pinselin, aspergillusone A 12-O-acetyl-AGI-B4 [30]. Screening for new bioactive metabolites from the marine-determined variety of *Aspergillus*, an *Aspergillus versicolor DJ013* separated from a coastal, Dongji Island, China. EtOAc separate resulted in identification and isolation of new furandione compounds, named asperfurandiones A and B [31]. Botryosphaerin were detached from the endophytic fungi *Botryosphaeria sp*. MHF associated with Maytenus hookeri. A compound CJ-14445 showed inhibition towards *Saccharomyces cervisiae, Candida albicans* and *Penicillium avellaneum* UC-4376 in correlation with nystatin which was utilized as a positive control [32] (**Figure 2**).

2.1 Bioactivities

Xanalteric acids I (38) and II (39) are the two new compounds which were segregated from the organism *Alternaria sp*., taken from leaves of the Mangrove plant *Sonneratiaceae,* gathered in Dong Zhai Gang Mangrove Garden on Hainan Island, China. Compounds 38 and 39 showed frail anti-microbial action against multidrug-resistant *S. aureus* with MIC estimations of 686.81–343.40 μM [34]. *Spicellum roseum* yielded the equivalent *trichothecene* as is delivered by the *Trichothecium roseum*. The compound demonstrated antimicrobial properties against specific yeasts of *Saccharomyces cerevisiae* and *Candida albicans* [35]. The absolute number of lignin from chosen white, soft and brown rot fungi were isolated. These outcomes have uncovered that, most elevated ligninolytic capacity was seen in *P. ostreatus, P. eryngii S. hirsutum* (white rot fungi), *C. puteana H. pinastri* (brown

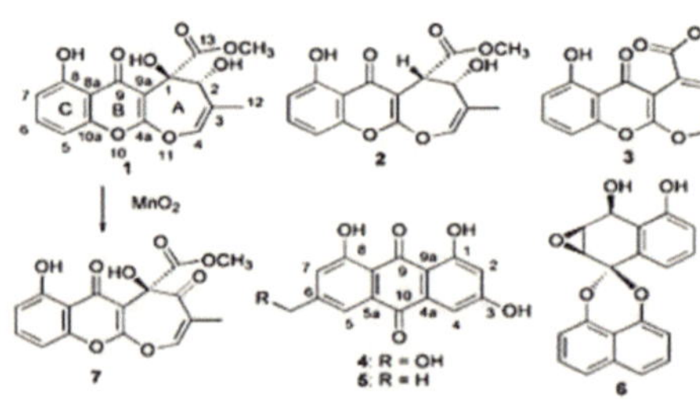

Figure 1.
Compounds 1–6 isolated from the endophytic fungus Microsphaeropsis sp. and 7 obtained by the oxidation of 1 [29].

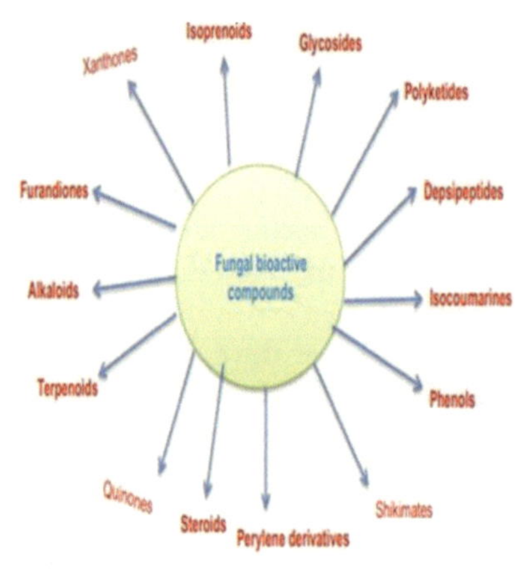

Figure 2.
Different types of fungal metabolites [33].

rot fungi) *F. oxysporum and B. dothidea* (soft rot fungi) [36]. The fungi recognized as *Neopestalotiopsis sp.,* active against *D. phaseolorum*. The outcomes feature that the endophytes are equipped for delivering compounds that might be utilized to control plant pathogens. The compound fumiquinone B is accounted for just because as an antifungal operator against *D. phaseolorum*, a significant plant pathogen around the world. This is additionally the first report of the production of fumiquinone B by the *Neopestalotiopsis* [37]. Fungi *M. albus* identified with *Cinnamomum zeylanicum*, recognized five classes of unstable compounds like alcohols, esters ketones, lipids and acids which smothered the action of pathogenic fungi, namely *Pythium ultimum, Phytophthora cinnamomi Rhizoctonia solani, Ustilago hordei, A.fumigates, Stagnosporanodorum, Sclerotinia sclerotiorum, Tapesia yallundae, F. solani, Cercospora beticola, C. albicans and Verticillum dahlia* [38]. The detached metabolite sclerotiorin from *Cephalotheca faveolata* had the capacity to incite apoptosis in malignant growth cells.

Sclerotiorin had apoptotic properties for colon malignant growth (HCT-116) cells by means of BAX and inactivated the BCL-2 proteins and further degrade the caspase-3 catalyst advancing apoptosis in dangerous cells [39]. Antibacterial action of the detached bioactive parts from endophytic growth *Phomopsis sp.* inside *Plumeria acutifolia* against the bacterial pathogens *E. coli, Klebsilla sp Pseudomonas sp., S. aureus, B. subtilis also, S. typhi* and it had no huge impact on *C. albicans* [40, 41]. *Awajanoran*, another dihydrobenzofuran derivative, was separated from an agar-culture of *Acremonium sp.* AWA16–1, which had been separated from ocean mud gathered at Awajishima Island in Japan. This compound restrained the development of A549 cells, the human lung adenocarcinoma cell line, with an IC50 estimation of 17 μg/ml, and furthermore demonstrated antimicrobial action [42]. R-135853 against different contagious strains and furthermore shows the MICs of R-135853 forthe strains utilized in vivo. R-135853 showed strong activity against *C. albicans, C. tropicalis, C. glabrata, C. neoformans and C. guilliermondii* with MICs varying from 0.016 to 0.5 g/ml [43].

3. Docking studies

A chain of 1-(1H-1,2,4-triazol-1-yl)- 2-(2,4-difluorophenyl)- 3-subbed 2-propanols (5a–5y) which are analogs of fluconazole, have been structured and integrated by means of Cu(I)- catalyzed azide–alkyne cycloaddition based on computational docking investigations to the dynamic site of the cytochrome P450 14α-demethylase

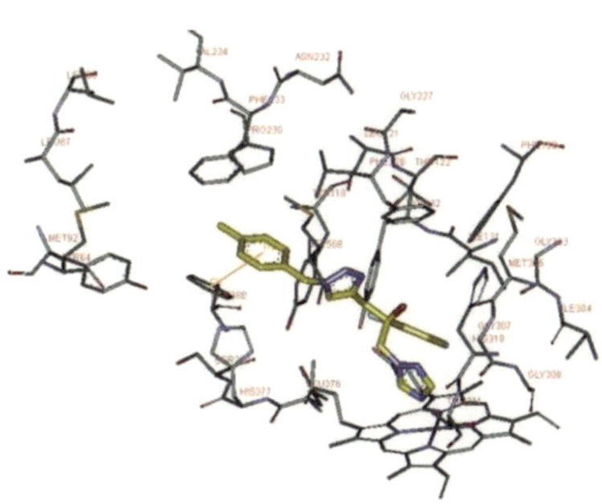

Figure 3.
Compounds binding geometry of the new inhibitor 5 l in the active site of CYP51 [44].

(CYP51). Target compounds were assessed against eight human pathogenic fungi in vitro. Compound 5 l demonstrated the best antifungal activity [44] (**Figure 3**).

Tyrosol, extracted from *P. chrysogenum* DXY-1, a marine fungi utilized as a QS inhibitor against *C. violaceum* and *P. aeruginosa*. The docking results show that tyrosol hinders the QS system of CviR in *C. violaceum* by binding to the DNA-binding domain and blocking the gene expression of pathogens [45] (**Figure 4**).

Three compounds (heptadecanoic acid, 16 methyl-, methyl ester; 9,12-octadecadienoic acid; cis-9-octadecenoic corrosive) identified and were screened against the skin cancer protein (Hsp90) by in-silico docking. The metabolites in two fungal strains of Hypocrea species were analyzed in GC–MS and the compound (Heptadecanoic corrosive, 16 methyl) indicated the best outcome against skin cancer protein [46] (**Figure 5**).

A 3D model of the cytochrome P450 14a-sterol demethylase of *C. albicans* (CA-CYP51) was built on the premise of the sequence homology with structure of the cytochrome P450 14a-sterol demethylases of M. tuberculosis (MT-CYP51). The model of CA-CYP51 was utilized to clarify the antifungal movement of a chain of 1,4-benzothiazine and 1,4-benzoxazine imidazole derivatives. All compounds receive comparable binding modes inside the catalytic site of CA-CYP51. These outcomes will be used to address the structure and synthesis of new strong antifungal compounds supplied with hostile to Candida action [47] (**Figure 6**).

Mannich bases of thiosemicarbazide is tested for anti-fungal activity. Docking of compounds was performed on the pdb structure of Lanosterol 14 α-demethylase (CYP51A1, P45014DM) utilizing Vlife MDS 3.5 as target. All incorporated atoms

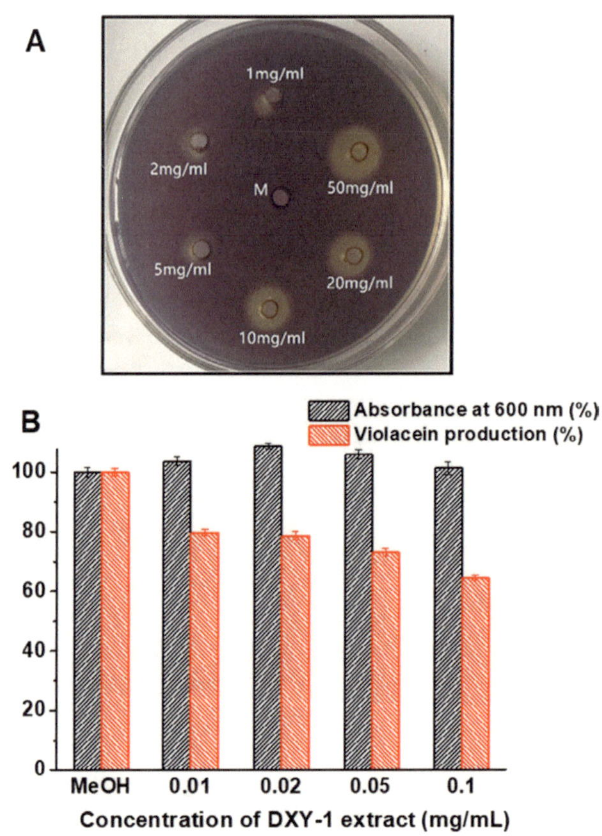

Figure 4.
Effects of tyrosol on the growth of C. violaceum CV026 and violacein production in C. violaceum [45].

DOI: http://dx.doi.org/10.5772/intechopen.94137

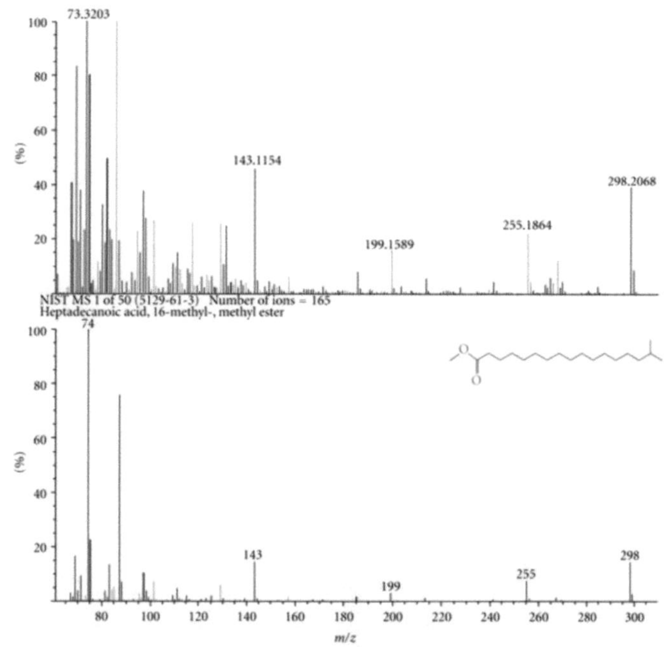

Figure 5.
GC–MS result of potential compound Heptadecanoic acid, 16 methyl derived from Hypocrea lixii TSK8 [46].

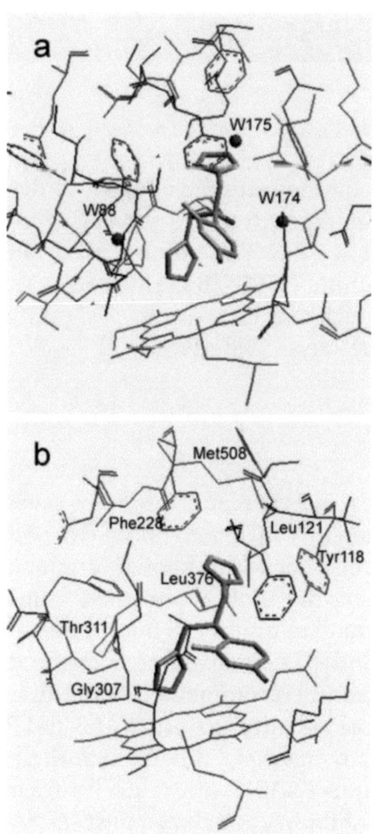

Figure 6.
Best docking solution of fluconazole into the catalytic site of CA-CYP51 [47].

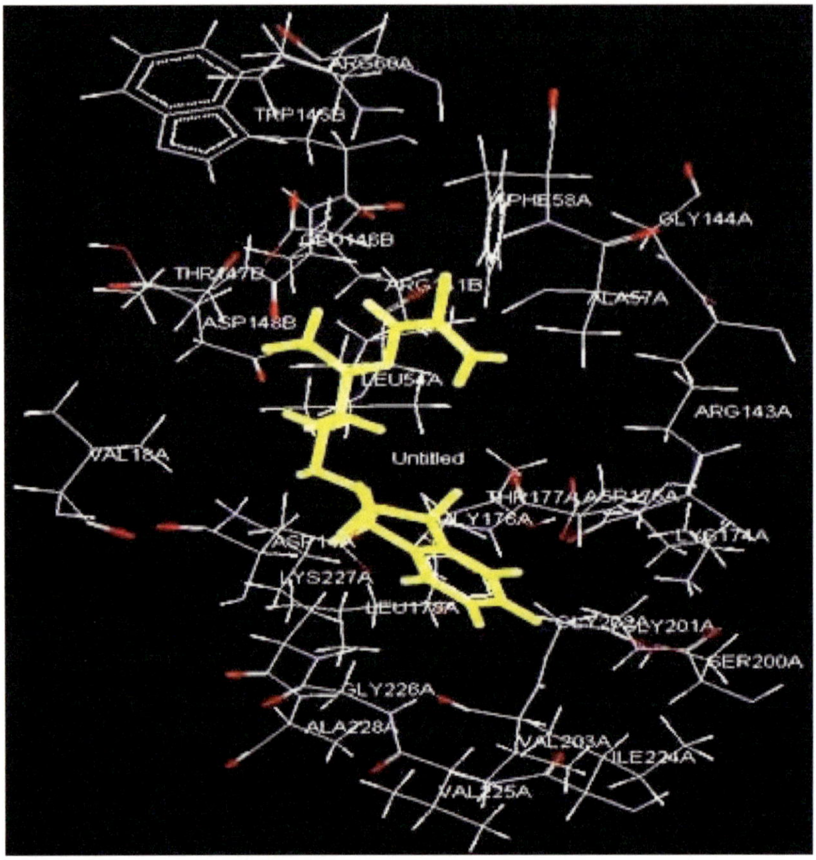

Figure 7.
Representative interactions shown by K_{20} with amino acid residues of CYP51A1, P45014DM [48].

were docked into a similar binding site. Docking study demonstrated a solid hydrophobicity between amino acids, such as Arganine (ARG141), Glutamine (GLU146), with hydrogen of aldehyde at 2.279. The amino acids included are Glycine GLY176A, Aspartine ASP175A, Threonine THR147B Lysine LYS227A, Phenyl alanine PHE58A and Arganine ARG141B which may be assuming a significant role in the specific binding of compounds with target [48] (**Figure 7**).

4. Recent discoveries

In this investigation, researchers scanned for new secondary metabolites from ocean inferred growth strain FKJ-0025 and found two new compounds, sarcopodinols A (1) and B (2), together with a known compound, SF-227. This is the principal report of secondary metabolites separated from family Sarcopodium. Cytotoxicity test utilizing human tumor cell lines, 1 demonstrated cytotoxicity against Jurkat cells. Eminently, 2 demonstrated cytotoxicity against HL-60, Jurkat, and Panc1 cells. These outcomes recommend that the absence of 5′-OH is the significant factor behind the lethality against HL-60 and Panc1 cells [49]. The novel Anthraquinone, 2-(dimethoxymethyl)- 1-hydroxyanthracene-9,10-dione, jointly with nine studied compounds (2–10), were taken from a marine derived fungi *A. versicolor*. 1 showed solid inhibitory activity against MRSA ATCC 43300 and MRSA CGMCC 12409 (with MIC estimations of 3.9 and 7.8 μg/mL separately) and moderate activity against analyzed strains of Vibrio. Molecular docking studies with

AmpC β-lactamase IV and topoisomerase indicated least binding interactions and supported antimicrobial movement of this compound is a novel compound merited expanding consideration as a source of antibacterial factor [50].

4.1 Antimicrobial agents

Antifungal peptides created by certain lactic acid bacteria strains have high potential for applications in expansive scope of nourishments. The component of peptides antifungal movement is identified with their properties, for example, low atomic weight, secondary structure, concentrations. The antifungal peptides were proposed to be utilized as bio-additives to decrease as well as supplant chemical preservatives [51]. White rot fungi that go under the division eumycota are heterogeneous gathering of fungi having ability to degrade a wide assortment of difficult compounds. Xenobiotic degradation may be due to non-specific enzymes. Manganese peroxidase, laccase, lignin peroxidase were explored seriously for the wide scope of xenobiotics. These organisms are having the ability to separate the lignin in wood without degrading cellulose, sometimes both cellulose and lignin will be degraded [52]. Nanotechnology for the creation of nanoparticles utilizing fungal cells is an ongoing phenomenon. Parasite like *Colletotrichum sp., A. clavatus, and Pestalotia sp.* have been utilized for improvement of nanoparticles against pathogenic microorganisms [33].

5. Conclusion

Bioinformatics has built up itself as a basic apparatus in target revelation. In silico pharmacology paradigm is progressing and presents a rich exhibit of chances that will help with expediating the revelation of new targets, and leads to discovery of compounds with biological activities. The drug design is based on analysis of structure of fungal species complexes. Various evaluations are found using quasi in vivo assay and pharmacokinetic analysis. For example, X-ray structures of *C. albicans* CYP51 complexes with posaconazole and VT-1161, providing a molecular mechanism for the potencies of these drugs against pathogens that are intrinsically resistant to fluconazole.

Future perspectives

Comparative structural analysis indicates the phylum-specific CYP51 features highlights that could coordinate future rational improvement of more productive expansive range antifungals. Basic assay normally focused on antimicrobial and antifungal activity. Viable and safe medications in the field on infections and malignant growth are unquestionably required. Subsequently, it is recommended to widen biological screens for the once in a while examined biological activities, which might be significant for the treatment of ceaseless illnesses.

Author details

Parthiban Brindha Devi* and Ridhanya Jayaseelan
Department of Bio Engineering, School of Engineering, Vels Institute of Science, Technology and Advanced Studies (VISTAS), Pallavaram, Chennai, Tamilnadu, India

*Address all correspondence to: pbrindhadevi@gmail.com

References

[1] Schueffler, Anja, and Timm Anke. "Fungal natural products in research and development." *Natural product reports* 31, no. 10 (2014): 1425-1448.

[2] Amend, Anthony, Gaetan Burgaud, Michael Cunliffe, Virginia P. Edgcomb, Cassandra L. Ettinger, M. H. Gutiérrez, Joseph Heitman et al. "Fungi in the marine environment: Open questions and unsolved problems." *MBio* 10, no. 2 (2019): e01189-18.

[3] Rateb, Mostafa E., and Rainer Ebel. "Secondary metabolites of fungi from marine habitats." *Natural product reports* 28, no. 2 (2011): 290-344.

[4] Hassett, Brandon T., Anne-Lise L. Ducluzeau, Roy E. Collins, and Rolf Gradinger. "Spatial distribution of aquatic marine fungi across the western Arctic and sub-arctic." *Environmental microbiology* 19, no. 2 (2017): 475-484.

[5] Molinski, Tadeusz F., Doralyn S. Dalisay, Sarah L. Lievens, and Jonel P. Saludes. "Drug development from marine natural products." *Nature reviews Drug discovery* 8, no. 1 (2009): 69.

[6] Butler, Mark S., Avril AB Robertson, and Matthew A. Cooper. "Natural product and natural product derived drugs in clinical trials." *Natural product reports* 31, no. 11 (2014): 1612-1661.

[7] PASSAES, Caroline P., and Asier SÁEZ-CIRIÓN. "HIV cure research: Advances and prospects. Virology, [sl], v. 454-455." (2014): 340-352.

[8] Wu, Bin, Gang Chen, Zhuo-gang Liu, and Yuhu Pei. "Two new alkaloids from a marine-derived fungus *Neosartorya fischeri*." *Records of Natural Products* 9, no. 3 (2015): 271.

[9] Wu, Bin, Jutta Wiese, Arlette Wenzel-Storjohann, Susan Malien, Rolf Schmaljohann, and Johannes F. Imhoff. "Engyodontochones, antibiotic polyketides from the marine fungus Engyodontium album Strain LF069." *Chemistry–A European Journal* 22, no. 22 (2016): 7452-7462.

[10] Gomes, Nelson GM, Florence Lefranc, Anake Kijjoa, and Robert Kiss. "Can some marine-derived fungal metabolites become actual anticancer agents?." *Marine Drugs* 13, no. 6 (2015): 3950-3991.

[11] Deshmukh, Sunil K., Ved Prakash, and Nihar Ranjan. "Marine fungi: A source of potential anticancer compounds." *Frontiers in microbiology* 8 (2018): 2536.

[12] Gladfelter, Amy S., Timothy Y. James, and Anthony S. Amend. "Marine fungi." *Current Biology* 29, no. 6 (2019): R191-R195.

[13] Bushley, Kathryn E., and B. Gillian Turgeon. "Phylogenomics reveals subfamilies of fungal nonribosomal peptide synthetases and their evolutionary relationships." *BMC evolutionary biology* 10, no. 1 (2010): 26.

[14] Richards, Thomas A., Meredith DM Jones, Guy Leonard, and David Bass. "Marine fungi: their ecology and molecular diversity." *Annual review of marine science* 4 (2012): 495-522.

[15] Wiese, Jutta, Birgit Ohlendorf, Martina Blümel, Rolf Schmaljohann, and Johannes F. Imhoff. "Phylogenetic identification of fungi isolated from the marine sponge Tethya aurantium and identification of their secondary metabolites." *Marine Drugs* 9, no. 4 (2011): 561-585.

[16] Bugni, Tim S., and Chris M. Ireland. "Marine-derived fungi: a chemically and biologically diverse group of microorganisms." *Natural Product Reports* 21, no. 1 (2004): 143-163.

[17] Imhoff, Johannes F., Antje Labes, and Jutta Wiese. "Bio-mining the microbial treasures of the ocean: new natural products." *Biotechnology advances* 29, no. 5 (2011): 468-482.

[18] Wang, Yan-Ting, Ya-Rong Xue, and Chang-Hong Liu. "A brief review of bioactive metabolites derived from deep-sea fungi." *Marine drugs* 13, no. 8 (2015): 4594-4616.

[19] Le Calvez, Thomas, Gaëtan Burgaud, Stéphane Mahé, Georges Barbier, and Philippe Vandenkoornhuyse. "Fungal diversity in deep-sea hydrothermal ecosystems." *Appl. Environ. Microbiol.* 75, no. 20 (2009): 6415-6421.

[20] Imhoff, Johannes F. "Natural products from marine fungi—Still an underrepresented resource." *Marine drugs* 14, no. 1 (2016): 19.

[21] Terstappen GC, Reggiani A. In silico research in drug discovery. Trends in pharmacological sciences. 2001 Jan 1;22(1):23-6.

[22] 52. Ekins S, Mestres J, Testa B. In silico pharmacology for drug discovery: applications to targets and beyond. British journal of pharmacology. 2007 Sep;152(1):21-37.

[23] 23.Zhang, Yapeng, Tianjiao Zhu, Yuchun Fang, Hongbing Liu, Qianqun Gu, and Weiming Zhu. "Carbonarones A and B, new bioactive γ-pyrone and α-pyridone derivatives from the marine-derived fungus Aspergillus carbonarius." *The Journal of antibiotics* 60, no. 2 (2007): 153.

[24] Zhang, Min, Wen-Liang Wang, Yu-Chun Fang, Tian-Jiao Zhu, Qian-Qun Gu, and Wei-Ming Zhu. "Cytotoxic alkaloids and antibiotic nordammarane triterpenoids from the marine-derived fungus Aspergillus sydowi." *Journal of natural products* 71, no. 6 (2008): 985-989.

[25] Scherlach, K.; Boettger, D.; Remme, N.; Hertweck, C. The chemistry and biology of cytochalasans. Nat. Prod. Rep. 2010, 27, 869-886.

[26] Masi, M.; Evidente, A.; Meyer, S.; Nicholson, J.; Munoz, A. Effect of strain and cultural conditions on the production of cytochalasin B by the potential mycoherbicide Pyrenophora semeniperda (Pleosporaceae, Pleosporales). Biocontrol. Sci. Technol. 2014, 24, 53-64.

[27] Skellam, E. The biosynthesis of cytochalasans. Nat. Prod. Rep. 2017, 34, 1252-1263.

[28] Masi, M.; Meyer, S.; Cimmino, A.; Clement, S.; Black, B.; Evidente, A. Pyrenophoric acids B and C, two new phytotoxic sesquiterpenoids produced by Pyrenophora semeniperda. J. Agric. Food Chem. 2014, 62, 10304-10311.

[29] Krohn, Karsten, Simeon F. Kouam, Guy M. Kuigoua, Hidayat Hussain, Stephan Cludius-Brandt, Ulrich Flörke, Tibor Kurtán et al. "Xanthones and Oxepino [2, 3-b] chromones from Three Endophytic Fungi." *Chemistry–A European Journal* 15, no. 44 (2009): 12121-12132.

[30] Song, Zhijun, Jieyu Gao, Jiansen Hu, Hongtao He, Pei Huang, Lixin Zhang, and Fuhang Song. "One new xanthenone from the marine-derived fungus Aspergillus versicolor MF160003." *Natural product research* (2019): 1-6.

[31] Ding, Lijian, Peng Xu, Te Li, Xiaojian Liao, Shan He, and Shihai Xu. "Asperfurandiones A and B, two antifungal furandione analogs from a marine-derived fungus Aspergillus versicolor." *Natural product research* 33, no. 23 (2019): 3404-3408.

[32] Souza, Jucimar Jorgeane de, Ivo José Curcino Vieira, Edson Rodrigues-Filho, and Raimundo Braz-Filho. "Terpenoids

from endophytic fungi." *Molecules* 16, no. 12 (2011): 10604-10618.

[33] Srivastava, Akhileshwar Kumar, and Israel Negev. "The role of fungus in bioactive compound production and nanotechnology." (2019).

[34] Kjer, Julia, Victor Wray, RuAngelie Edrada-Ebel, Rainer Ebel, Alexander Pretsch, Wenhan Lin, and Peter Proksch. "Xanalteric acids I and II and related phenolic compounds from an endophytic Alternaria sp. isolated from the mangrove plant *Sonneratia alba*." *Journal of natural products* 72, no. 11 (2009): 2053-2057.

[35] Langley, P., A. Shuttleworth, P. J. Sidebottom, S. K. Wrigley, and P. J. Fisher. "A trichothecene from Spicellum roseum." *Mycological research* 94, no. 5 (1990): 705-706.

[36] Sista Kameshwar, Ayyappa Kumar, and Wensheng Qin. "Comparative study of genome-wide plant biomass-degrading CAZymes in white rot, brown rot and soft rot fungi." *Mycology* 9, no. 2 (2018): 93-105.

[37] Grigoletto, Diana Fortkamp, Ana Maria Lima Correia, Wolf-Rainer Abraham, Andre Rodrigues, Marco Antonio Assis, Antonio Gilberto Ferreira, Michelli Massaroli, and Simone Possedente de Lira. "Secondary metabolites produced by endophytic fungi: novel antifungal activity of fumiquinone B." *Acta Scientiarum. Biological Sciences* 41 (2019): e48785-e48785.

[38] Harper, J.K., Ford, E.J., Strobel, G.A., Arif, A., Grant, D.M., Porco, J., et al., 2003. Pestacin: a 1,3,-dihydro isobenofuran from Pestalotipsis microspora possessing antioxidant and antimycotic activities. Tetrahedron 59, 2471_2476.

[39] Santiago, C., Chris, F., Murray, H.G.M., Juriyati, J., Jacinta, S., 2012. Cytotoxic and antifungal activities of 5-hydroxyramulosin, a compound produced by an endophytic fungus isolated from Cinnamomum mollissimum. Evid-Based Compl Alt. Med. 1_6.

[40] Tayung, K., Barik, B.P., Jha, D.K., Deka, D.C., 2011. Identification and characterization of antimicrobial metabolite from an endophytic fungus, *Fusarium solani* isolated from bark of Himalayan yew. Mycosphere 2, 203_213.

[41] Nithya, K., Muthumary, J., 2010. Secondary metabolite from Phomopsis sp. isolated from *Plumeria acutifolia* Poiret. Recent Res. Sci. Technol. 2, 99_103.

[42] Jang, Jae-Hyuk, Kaneo Kanoh, Kyoko Adachi, and Yoshikazu Shizuri. "New dihydrobenzofuran derivative, awajanoran, from marine-derived Acremonium sp. AWA16-1." *The Journal of antibiotics* 59, no. 7 (2006): 428.

[43] Fukuoka, Takashi, Shogo Kuwahara, Yasuki Kamai, Masayo Kakuta, and Takahiro Shibayama. "Antifungal Activities of R-135853."

[44] Zou, Yan, Qingjie Zhao, Jun Liao, Honggang Hu, Shichong Yu, Xiaoyun Chai, Mingjuan Xu, and Qiuye Wu. "New triazole derivatives as antifungal agents: Synthesis via click reaction, in vitro evaluation and molecular docking studies." *Bioorganic & medicinal chemistry letters* 22, no. 8 (2012): 2959-2962.

[45] Chang A, Sun S, Li L, Dai X, Li H, He Q, Zhu H. Tyrosol from marine Fungi, a novel Quorum sensing inhibitor against Chromobacterium violaceum and *Pseudomonas aeruginosa*. Bioorganic chemistry. 2019 Oct 1;91:103140.

[46] Kandasamy S, Sahu SK, Kandasamy K. In Silico studies on fungal metabolite against skin cancer

protein (4, 5-Diarylisoxazole HSP90 Chaperone). ISRN dermatology. 2012;2012.

[47] Macchiarulo, Antonio, Gabriele Costantino, Daniele Fringuelli, Anna Vecchiarelli, Fausto Schiaffella, and Renata Fringuelli. "1, 4-Benzothiazine and 1, 4-benzoxazine imidazole derivatives with antifungal activity: a docking study." *Bioorganic & medicinal chemistry* 10, no. 11 (2002): 3415-3423.

[48] Pishawikar, Sachin A., and Harinath N. More. "Synthesis, docking and in-vitro screening of mannich bases of thiosemicarbazide for anti-fungal activity." *Arabian Journal of Chemistry* 10 (2017): S2714-S2722.

[49] Matsuo, Hirotaka, Kenichi Nonaka, Yuriko Nagano, Akinori Yabuki, Katsunori Fujikura, Yōko Takahashi, Satoshi Ōmura, and Takuji Nakashima. "New metabolites, sarcopodinols A and B, isolated from deep-sea derived fungal strain Sarcopodium sp. FKJ-0025." *Bioscience, biotechnology, and biochemistry* 82, no. 8 (2018): 1323-1326.

[50] Wang, Weiyi, Ruixuan Chen, Zhuhua Luo, Wei Wang, and Jianming Chen. "Antimicrobial activity and molecular docking studies of a novel anthraquinone from a marine-derived fungus Aspergillus versicolor." *Natural product research* 32, no. 5 (2018): 558-563.

[51] Muhialdin, B. J., H. L. Algboory, N. K. Mohammed, H. Kadum, A. S. M. Hussin, N. Saari, and Z. Hassan. "Discovery and Development of Novel Anti-fungal Peptides Against Food-spoiling Fungi." *Current drug discovery technologies* (2019).

[52] Yadav, Ajar Nath, Sangram Singh, Shashank Mishra, and Arti Gupta, eds. *Recent Advancement in White Biotechnology Through Fungi: Volume 3: Perspective for Sustainable Environments*. Springer Nature, 2019.

Chapter 7

Studies on Histamine H2-Receptor Antagonists by Using Density Functional Theory

Kodakkat Parambil Safna Hussan, Indulekha Jayarajan Jithin Raj, Sailaja Urpayil and Mohamed Shahin Thayyil

Abstract

Density functional theory (DFT) is a quantum mechanical approach used to investigate the electronic structure (principally the ground state) of many-body systems, in particular atoms, molecules, and the condensed phases. In this work, we have used DFT/B3LYP/6-31+G(d) level of theory to get insight into the molecular geometry and thermochemical properties of histamine H2-receptor antagonists. Histamine H2-receptor antagonists or H2 blockers are a group of pharmaceutical ingredients that reduce the amount of acid produced by the cells in the lining of the stomach. The potential H2 blockers include cimetidine, famotidine, nizatidine, and ranitidine. The detailed theoretical investigation on the listed H2 blockers in terms of their thermochemical parameters and global descriptive parameters revealed that, though famotidine is the best among them with highest Gibbs free energy, nizatidine showed higher biological activity with high softness, low hardness, and high electrophilicity index. The theoretical vibrational spectra of these four Histamine H2-receptor antagonists were analyzed and the infrared spectra of nizatidine was compared with the experimental IR spectra, and found to be good agreement with the experimental values. Further, frontier molecular orbitals especially the highest occupied molecular orbital (HOMO) and the lowest unoccupied molecular orbital (LUMO) were determined and the activation energy of the selected samples were calculated. In addition to this, the amorphisation technique were employed to enhance the solubility and bio availability of the best biologically active H2 blocker nizatidine using broadband dielectric spectroscopy.

Keywords: histamine H2-receptor antagonists, density functional theory, molecular orbitals

1. Introduction

The branch of computational chemistry is identified to be one of the nascent applications of technological growth within chemistry. Within this branch, different algorithms are introduced through incorporating aspects of theoretical chemistry for identifying and predicting chemical properties of compounds. Analyzing the results obtained from computational chemistry it was fascinating to note that the theoretical results provide information with same quality of the data obtained through conducting experiments. With the required level of availability of variables or data, it helps in describing various unobserved chemical phenomena [1]. Computational chemistry is identified to be one of the major components identified to be included in the process of making new chemical products. The use of this technology provides increased efficiency of the drug introduced through analyzing the nature of the particular receptor site. The role of organic chemists is followed by attempting to synthesize the proposed structure of the chemical components, which is occasionally tested by biochemists. This set of actions is iterated by analyzing experimental results after obtaining feedback on the same. The aspect of the feed back provides suggestions for effectively increasing the quality of molecules.

Various tools used by computational chemistry starting from molecular mechanics to higher quantum mechanical calculations including Hartree Fock method, density functional methods & ab initio calculations. The balls and springs model of molecules is identified to be included within molecular mechanics [2]. The element of quantum mechanics is introduced within the ab initio aspect through treating the same with the Schrödinger Equation [3]. Semi-empirical methods are identified to include Hartree-Fock theory in a more simplified version along with empirical corrections resulting in increased performance [4]. DFT or Density Function Theory uses electron density function irrespective of the wave function. The electron density function is also identified as charge density or just merely electron density. Two of the Hohenberg-Kohn theorems which describe that the ground state property of atom or molecule is identified by its electron density function and the energy produced by trial electron density should be either greater than or equal to its true and valid energy, are the main constituents of density functional theory [5]. The Kohn - Sham approach, on the other hand, is identified to analyze the level of variations made by a system through considering an ideal system that is comprised of non-interacting electrons [3]. Through reducing the energy along with Kohn-Sham orbitals, the Kohn-Sham equations can be derived from the energy equation [6, 7].

Experiment and theory are identified to be the major components for the functioning of science and almost all of its disciplines. Hence, one without the other won't be able to effectively assist in the creation of scientific breakthroughs. A theory without experimental data to support it is regarded as a hypothesis, while experiments without theory will not provide a degree of finiteness to it. In the field of science, the advent of the computational facility is identified to provide increased support for such experimental needs. Focusing on the branch of chemistry, computational chemistry is identified to effectively assist in various experimental chores [1]. The major reason for the success of computational chemistry was the chance provided for skipping over the tedious and hazardous chemical experimentation with the help of computer simulation.

Here in this work structural properties along with the reactivity, energy, vibrational properties and frontier molecular orbitals of histamine H2-receptor antagonists (cimetidine, famotidine, nizatidine and ranitidine), are investigated using Density functional theory [4]. H2 blockers are a group of medicines that reduce the amount of acid produced by the cells in the lining of the stomach and are used to treat duodenal ulcers, gastric ulcers and Zollinger-Ellison disease [8]. They are also called 'histamine H2-receptor antagonists' but are commonly called H2 blockers. The H2 blockers compete with histamine for H2 receptors on the stomach's parietal cells and thereby depress the production of hydrochloric acid. They are rapidly absorbed and will reach peak blood levels in 1 to 3 hours. Acid-suppression lasts several hours thereafter and permits peptic ulcers to heal over a few weeks. It also counteracts the corrosive effects of acid, which refluxes into the esophagus (food pipe) and causes heartburn. Though histamine H2 blockers inhibit the action of histamine on gastric H2 receptors thereby decreasing gastric acidity, they were considered a breakthrough in the treatment of peptic ulcer disease but it is used as non-NSAID ulcers, and control severe esophagitis. There are four H2 blockers available by prescription: cimetidine, ranitidine, nizatidine and famotidine [9]. But we are unaware about the chemical and biological activities of these H2 blockers and information are less to claim best among the four. This work is an attempt to get an insight to the structural and thermochemical properties and parameters such as Gibbs free energy, enthalpy and entropy, and stability of the four selected H2 blockers and to find out which molecule is comparatively active; chemically as well as biologically. Further we have included the molecular dynamics of the best one among the four H2 blockers to enhance its solubility by amorphosizing the sample by quench cooling technique, though such study is out of focus of this chapter.

2. Materials and method

2.1 Materials

The input structures the drugs; cimetidine (PubChem: 3033637); famotidine (PubChem: 2756); nizatidine (PubChem: 5702160); ranitidine (PubChem: 3001055) were taken from the PubChem database [10], which are in sdf (Standard Data File) format and were converted to GJF (Gaussian Job File) input files using the application Open Babel [11].

2.2 Computational methodology

All the quantum calculations have been performed by density functional theory using a Gaussian 09 software package [12]. The initial geometries chosen for calculation was taken from the PubChem database and optimized with DFT/B3LYP/6-31 + G(d) level of the theory [6]. The B3LYP is Becke's three-parameter practical hybrid methods that add the exchange and electronic correlation terms in DFT, including the Lee, Yang Parr (LYP) functional. The optimized geometry was used for the calculations of harmonic vibrational frequencies at the DFT/B3LYP/6-31 + G(d) method, it also helps to ensure the systems to be local minimum number imaginary vibration frequencies. The thermochemical properties [13–15] like, hardness (η), softness (S), chemical potential (μ), electronegativity (χ) and electrophilicity index (ω), were calculated using Koopman's theorem for closed-shell compounds. Electrostatic potential analysis has also been made to identify the mapping surface of drugs. The thermo chemical properties of the selected molecules were calculated from electronic energy, the equilibrium geometry and the vibrational frequencies.

3. Results and discussion

3.1 Molecular geometry

All four histamine H2 receptor antagonists: cimetidine, famotidine, nizatidine, and ranitidine were optimized using DFT method using B3LYP/6-31 + G(d) level of theory. Optimized geometry parameters of the four samples were listed out in the supplementary material for reference. The optimized structure of four H2 blockers were depicted in **Figure 1** [16–18].

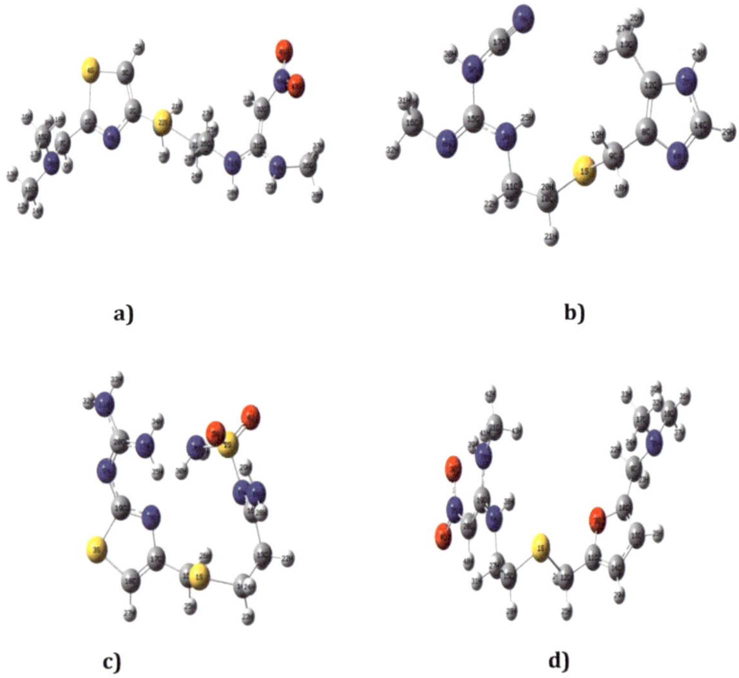

Figure 1.
Optimized molecular structures of Histamine H2 receptor antagonist using the B3LYP/6-31 + G (d) basis set. (a) nizatidine, (b) cimetidine, (c) famotidine and (d) ranitidine.

3.2 Vibrational analysis

Infrared (IR) spectroscopy refers the analysis of interaction of infrared radiation with a molecule. IR spectra of nizatidine obtained from DFT method using B3LYP/6-31 + G(d) level of theory (in **Figure 2(a)**) is compared with the experimental IR spectra (in **Figure 2(b)**) and their assignments were tabulated in **Table 1**.

From the comparison of IR spectra of nizatidine it is clear that, the computed vibrational results were in good agreement with the experimental spectra. IR spectra of cimetidine, famotidine and ranitidine are also generated using DFT method using B3LYP/6-31 + G(d) level of theory and shown in **Figures 3–5.**

The vibration at 3109 cm^{-1} shows the presence of N-H bond. The C-H band is present at 1741 for bending mode of vibration. The vibration band around 1435 and 1462 cm^{-1} are due to C-H scissor vibration. The bands due to C-N stretching are appeared at 1300 and 1255 cm^{-1}. The band due to C-C skeleton vibration are appeared at 544 and 508 cm^{-1}.

The band due to asymmetric NH_2 stretching vibration appears at 3336 cm^{-1} in the vibrational spectra of famotidine. The vibration band around 1696 and 1664 cm^{-1} are due to C=N stretching. The vibration at 1088 cm^{-1} shows the presence of C-N bond. The N-H band is present at 832 cm^{-1} for out of plain bending mode of vibration.

Spectral analysis of ranitidine shows a vibration at 3442 cm^{-1} and it is due to the presence of N-H bond. The C=C band is present at 1660 and 1588 cm^{-1} for stretching mode of vibration. The band due to NO_2 stretching is appeared at 1390 cm^{-1}. The vibration band around 1264 and 1174 cm^{-1} are due to C-N stretching.

3.3 Thermo-chemical properties

The reaction parameters of the four Histamine H2-receptor antagonists were calculated and tabulated below in **Table 2**.

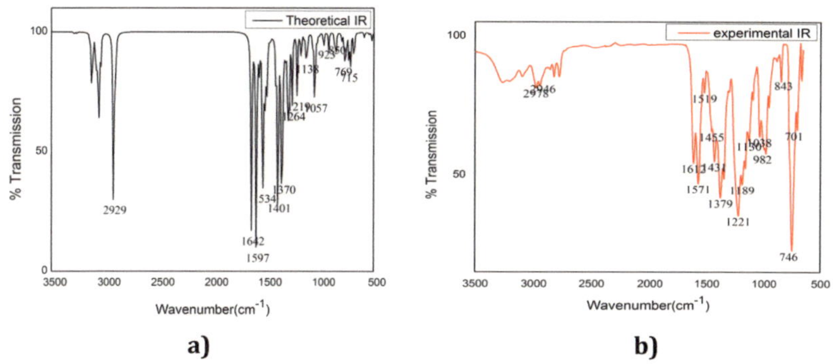

Figure 2.
Theoretical (DFT generated) IR spectra (a); experimental IR spectra (b) of nizatidine.

Experimental IR	DFT IR	Assignments
2978	2929	Asymmetric C-H stretching vibration
2946		
1612	1642	C-H vibration (overtone)
1571	1597	C=C stretching vibration
1519	1534	
1455	1401	Asymmetric C-H deformation vibration
1431		
1379	1370	Symmetric C-H deformation vibration
1221	1264	C-N stretching vibrations
1189	1219	
1130	1138	C-H sym. Deformation vibration
1038	1057	C-N stretching vibration
982	923	
843	850	C-H out-of-plane deformation vibration
746	769	C-C skeleton vibration (rocking)
701	715	CH3-metal groups due to CH2 rocking vibration

Table 1.
Vibrational analysis of nizatidine by experimental and theoretical obtained from DFT method using B3LYP/6-31 + G(d) level of theory.

By calculating reaction parameters of histamine H2 receptor antagonist it was found that famotidine is having high free energy, zero-point energy, enthalpy and low entropy. If the Gibbs free energy is higher the solubility will be higher i.e. famotidine having higher solubility. Nizatidine exhibits higher entropy value with less energy indicating that it has higher degree of freedom to be active. Cimetidine is less potent and having low solubility. If nizatidine get a small perturbation in terms of thermal energy it will be in full mode to be active for its specified task.

3.4 Frontier molecular orbital analysis

Both the energies of HOMO (Highest Occupied Molecular Orbitals) and LUMO (Lowest Unoccupied Molecular Orbitals) are identified. The chemical reactivity of

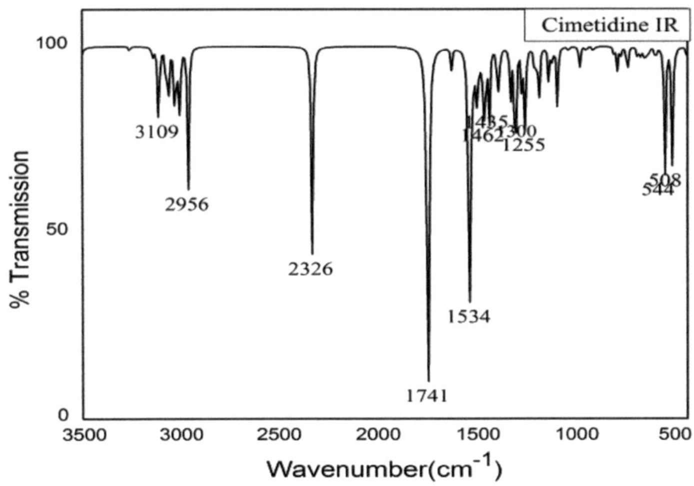

Figure 3.
Theoretical IR spectra of cimetidine using DFT/B3LYP/6-31 + G(d) level of theory.

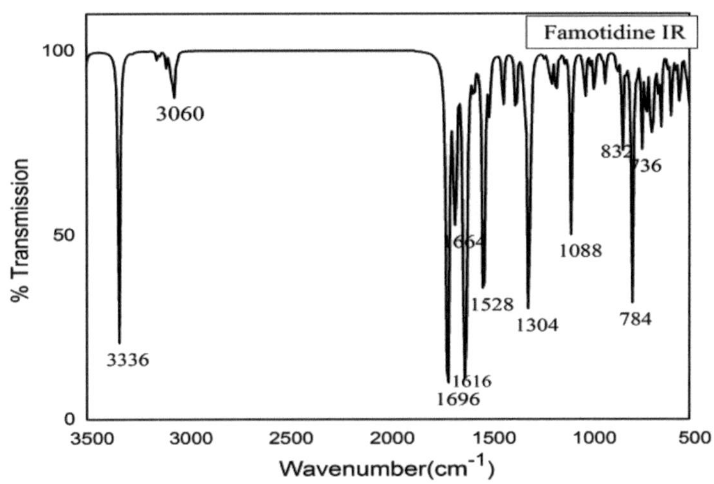

Figure 4.
Theoretical IR spectra of famotidine DFT/B3LYP/6-31 + G(d) level of theory.

a particular molecule can be determined from their energy gap and eigen values. In addition to being called the frontier orbitals, both HOMO and LUMO are identified to be effectively included within the study regarding charge transfer complex formation reactions [13]. HOMO is identified to represent the ability to be an electron donor through giving an electron, while LUMO, on the other hand, and focuses on the method of gaining electron through being an electron acceptor [14]. The wave function is identified to describe the process of electron absorption as the transition from the ground state to the next excited state. This process is further understood as the excitation of one electron from the highest occupied molecular orbital to the lowest level of an unoccupied molecular orbital. The element of energy gap within both HOMO and LUMO is identified as the parameter describing molecular transport properties [15]. The aspect of electron conductivity also can be understood through the measure of HOMO – LUMO gap along with molecular stability with a large gap denoting higher stability. Hence, the molecular orbitals of all four selected H2 blockers were generated and visualized using DFT, and these molecular orbitals

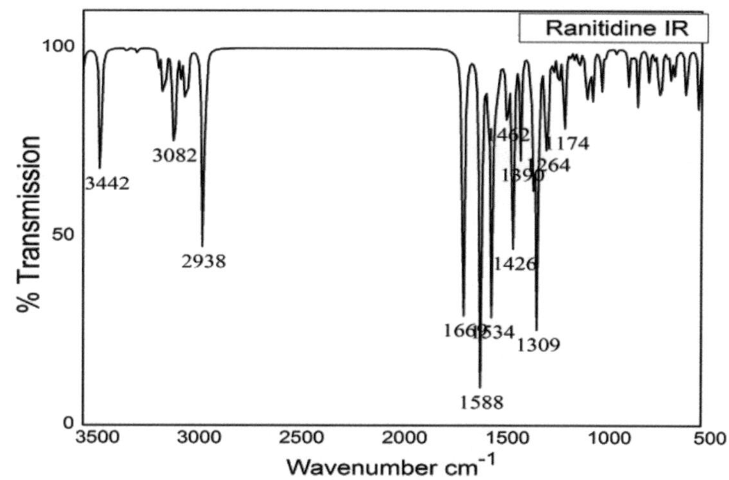

Figure 5.
Theoretical IR spectra of ranitidine DFT/B3LYP/6-31 + G(d) level of theory.

Sample	Molecular Mass (amu)	Zero point Energy (10^9 kJ/mol)	Enthalpy (10^9 kJ/mol)	Entropy (Cal/mol)	Gibbs Free Energy (10^9 kJ/mol)
Nizatidine	331.114	−4.43	−4.43	177.061	−4.43
Cimetidine	252.116	−2.93	−2.93	151.938	−2.93
Famotidine	337.045	−5.36	−5.36	153.901	−5.36
Ranitidine	314.141	−3.54	−3.54	172.629	−3.54

Table 2.
The reaction parameters of Histamine H2 receptor antagonist.

were shown in **Figure 6** (the positive phase is represented in red and the negative one in green).

The possible transitions exhibited by nizatidine and famotidine is π to $\pi*$ transition while cimetidine showed π to π transition and ranitidine exhibited a $\pi*$ to π transition. The least energy required must be for π to $\pi*$ transition and this may be the reason for high reactivity of nizatidine.

The HOMO, LUMO energies of the selected samples were calculated and tabulated below in **Table 3**.

The difference between HOMO and LUMO energy levels directly gives the band gap or energy gap of the compound. The higher the energy gap lower will be the reactivity of the molecule. Comparing the orbital energy parameters of histamine H2 receptor antagonist, nizatidine is found to be having lower energy gap, which shows that nizatidine is more chemically reactive than others. At the same time cimetidine has high energy gap indicating its less reactivity. So, we can infer that nizatidine is the most biologically active API while cimetidine is the least among the H2 blockers.

3.5 Global descriptive parameters

The global parameters are identified to have a larger role to play within the comparison of the behaviors of different compounds and their level of reactivity. A global descriptive parameter is identified to provide the description of the

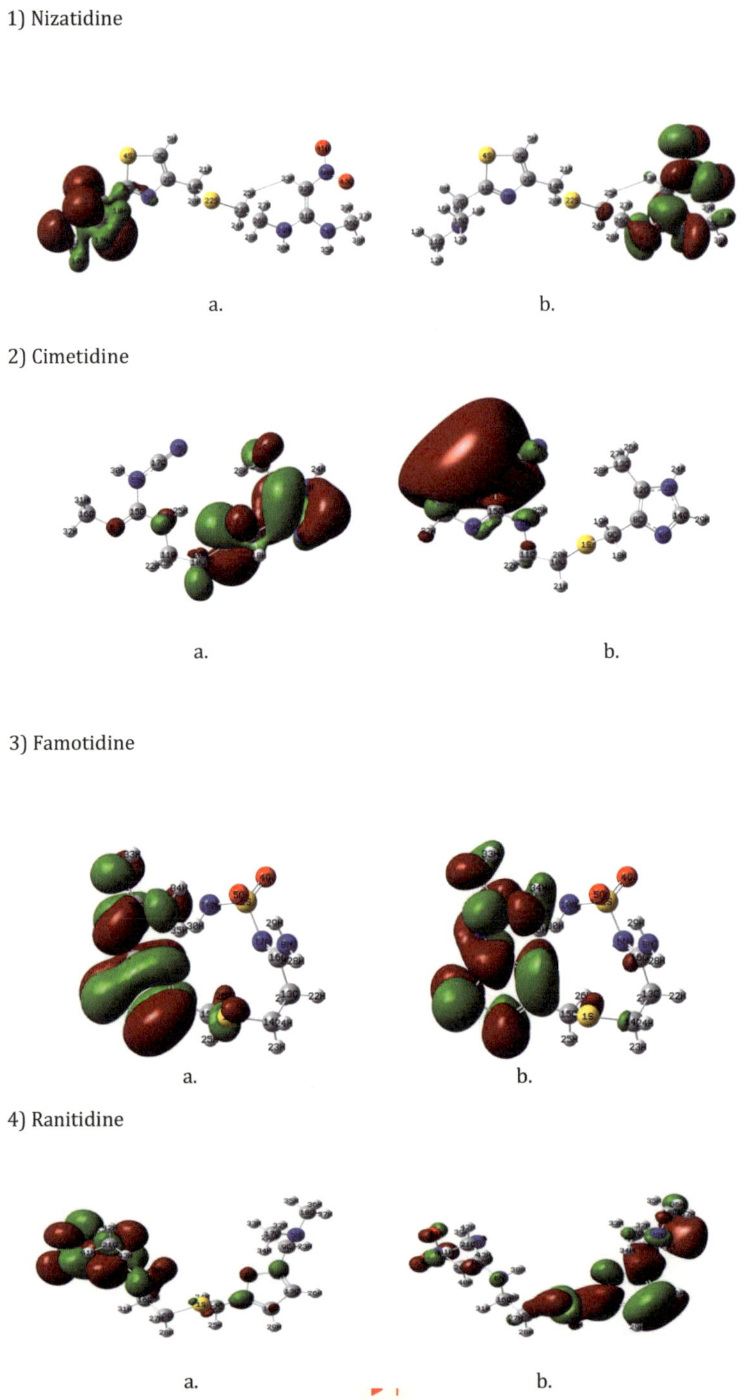

Figure 6.
Molecular orbitals of Histamine H2 receptor antagonist using the B3LYP/6-31 + G (d) basis set.
(1) a. HOMO Energy =- 6.209 eV, b. LUMO Energy = - 1.650 eV; (2) a. HOMO Energy = -6.052 eV, b. LUMO Energy = -0.475 eV; (3) a. HOMO Energy =- 5.755 eV, b. LUMO Energy = - 0.957 eV; (4) a. HOMO Energy = -6.114 eV, b. LUMO Energy = -1.439 eV.

connection between the chemical reactivity of the molecule along with the range of sensitiveness exhibited to the various external conditions. Various aspects such as chemical potential, chemical hardness, electro negativity, electrophilicity, and

Sample	E_{HOMO} (eV)	E_{LUMO} (eV)	ΔE (eV)
Nizatidine	−6.209	−1.650	4.559
Cimetidine	−6.052	−0.475	5.577
Famotidine	−5.755	−0.957	4.798
Ranitidine	−6.114	−1.439	4.675

Table 3.
Orbital energy parameters of studied compounds using DFT/B3LYP/6-31 + G (d) level of theory.

softness are contained within the global descriptive parameters. These quantities correspond to the linear responses of the electron density with respect to the changes in the external potential and number of electrons [13]. The aspect of chemical hardness (η) can be understood as the resistance introduced by elements towards deformation or even polarization of the electron cloud of the element which is introduced through following chemical reactions conducted upon the same. Chemical softness (s), on the contrary to the chemical hardness, is identified to provide a measure of the capacity of the molecule for receiving electrons [14]. Through analyzing this case by considering the aspect of the HOMO – LUMO gap, a hard element is identified to have a larger HOMO – LUMO gap compared to a softer element. As the aspect of electro negativity (χ) describes the ability of the molecule for attracting electrons and reaching equalization much more quickly, it is identified to introduce low reactivity. The tendency for an electron to escape from an equilibrium state is referred to as chemical potential while the strength of electrophilies of elements is identified through electrophilicity indices.

Koopmans' theorem states that in closed-shell Hartree–Fock theory, the first ionization energy of a molecular system is equal to the negative of the orbital energy of the highest occupied molecular orbital (HOMO) i.e., Koopmans' theorem equates the energy of the HOMO with the negative of the ionization potential [19]. The global properties were calculated by using equations [12, 13, 20].

$$\text{Ionization potential}\,(\text{IP}) \approx -\text{E}_{\text{HOMO}} \tag{1}$$

$$\text{Electron affinity}\,(\text{EA}) \approx -\text{E}_{\text{LUMO}} \tag{2}$$

where E_{HOMO} is the energy of HOMO and E_{LUMO} is the energy of LUMO.

$$\text{Hardness}\,(\eta) \approx \frac{IP - EA}{2.} \tag{3}$$

$$\text{Electronegativity}\,(\chi) \approx \frac{IP + EA}{2} \tag{4}$$

$$\text{Softness}\,(\text{S}) \approx \frac{1}{2\eta} \tag{5}$$

$$\text{Chemical potential}\,(\mu) \approx -\chi \tag{6}$$

$$\text{Electrophilicity index}\,(\omega) \approx \frac{\mu^2}{2\eta} \tag{7}$$

The Global descriptive parameters of the four histamine H2 receptor antagonists were calculated and tabulated below in **Table 4**.

Sample	IP (Ionization potential)	EA (Electron affinity)	χ (Electronegativity)	μ (Chemical potential)	ω (Electrophilicity index)	η (Hardness)	S (Softness)
Nizatidine	6.209	1.65	3.929	−3.929	3.387	2.279	0.219
Cimetidine	6.052	0.475	3.264	−3.264	1.91	2.789	0.179
Famotidine	5.755	0.957	3.356	−3.356	2.348	2.399	0.208
Ranitidine	6.114	1.439	3.776	−3.776	3.051	2.338	0.214

Table 4.
Global descriptors of studied compounds using DFT/B3LYP/6-31 + G (d) level of theory.

Comparing the global descriptive parameters of histamine H2 receptor antagonist, nizatidine is found to be having higher softness, ionization potential, electron affinity, chemical potential and lower hardness, which shows that nizatidine is less stable and chemically more reactive. A higher value of electrophilicity index indicates its high biological activity. In case of stability reactivity and biological activity, ranitidine comes next to nizatidine and among them, cimetidine is more stable and having lower biological activity.

3.6 Molecular dynamics

The theoretical studies revealed that nizatidine is highly stable and biological active molecule among the four histamine H2 receptor antagonists. But the value of Gibbs free energy emphasis that the solubility of nizatidine is less. The possible solution to enhance the solubility and bioavailability of the pharmaceutical drug is amorphisation of its crystalline counterpart. We have already reported the molecular dynamics of nizatidine in its glassy and supercooled liquid state using broadband dielectric spectroscopy [21]. The dielectric measurements of nizatidine were performed from 123.15 K to 373.15 K by quench cooling the sample. However, the sample does not crystallize during cooling from the melting temperature. Then the measured dielectric loss spectra (i.e., imaginary part of dielectric permittivity ε" plotted as a function of frequency f) are shown **Figure** 7.

The dielectric measurements revealed that the sample nizatidine is a good glass former with glass transition temperature Tg around 282.09 K with steepness index 91 without showing any recrystalisation tendency during heating and cooling. The steepness index is the measure of the non-Arrhenius character of the temperature dependence of the α-relaxation times. In contrast to strong liquids (m = 16), fragile glass-forming materials (m = 200) show a fast change in its viscosity (relaxation time) as it approaches the glass transition temperature. The knowledge whether a glass former is strong or fragile seems to be essential in case of choosing the best temperature condition for storing an amorphous pharmaceutical where the structural relaxation

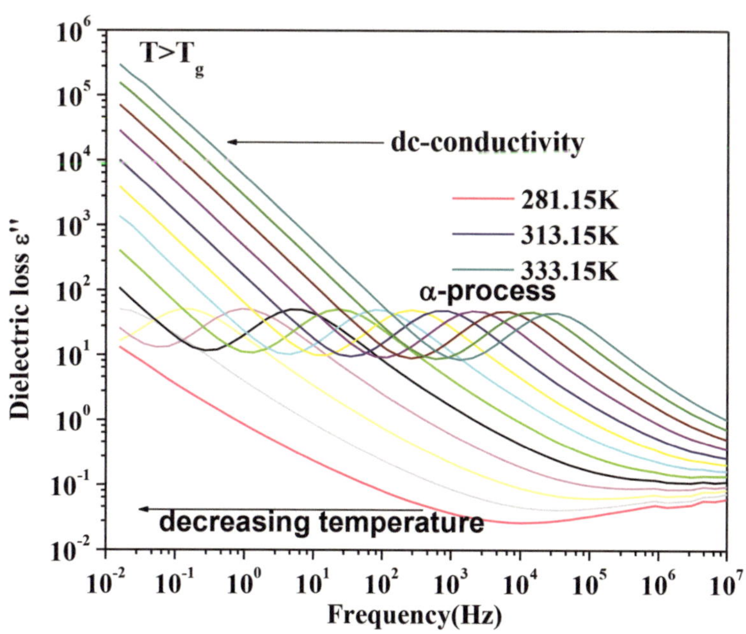

Figure 7.
Dielectric loss curves obtained for nizatidine in the supercooled liquid state [21].

is closely connected to crystallization process [22]. And it is found that nizatidine is stable over the measured temperature range up to 307.15 K. Of course, the dielectric studies is only giving an indication on the molecular mobility, for detailed information regarding the molecular mobility of nizatidine in glassy and supercooled liquid state refer paper published by Sailaja et al. [21].

4. Conclusions

Density functional theory calculation using DFT/B3LYP/6-31 + G (d) level of theory has been performed for four histamine H2 receptor antagonists, cimetidine, famotidine, nizatidine, and ranitidine with the help of Gaussian software. Vibrational analysis (IR) of four histamine H2 receptor antagonists has been generated by using DFT. Generated vibrational results of nizatidine were compared with the experimental result and the computed vibrational results found to be in good agreement with the experimental result. From thermochemical parameters of histamine H2 receptor antagonist, it was found that famotidine is having superior thermodynamics parameters among the four with high free energy, zero-point energy, enthalpy and low entropy. Comparing the global descriptive parameters of histamine H2 receptor antagonist, nizatidine is found to be having higher softness, ionization potential, electron affinity, chemical potential and lower hardness, which shows that it is more stable and chemically reactive. Higher value of electrophilicity index indicates its high biological activity. Nizatidine is found to be having lower energy gap, which shows that nizatidine is more chemically reactive. In case of stability, reactivity and biological activity ranitidine comes next to nizatidine and among them, cimetidine is less stable and having lower biological activity. At the same time, the Gibb's free energy revealed that the solubility of nizatidine is not sufficient to have adequate bioavailability. Finally, we could amorphousize nizatidine by quench cooling technique and found that it stable in amorphous state without showing any recrystallization tendency during super cooling and the subsequent heating in the metastable state. Nizatidine has a glass transition temperature around 282.1 K and was found to be stable over the measured temperature range up to 307 K.

Acknowledgments

One of the authors I. J. Jithin Raj is grateful to Mr. Mubarak N, Head, Department of Physics Kottakkal Farook Arts and Science College, Ashna Poulose Department of Physics, University of Calicut for the help and co-operation during this work. This research did not receive any specific grant from funding agencies in the public, commercial, or not-for-profit sectors.

Conflict of interest

The authors declare no conflict of interest.

Author details

Kodakkat Parambil Safna Hussan[1*], Indulekha Jayarajan Jithin Raj[2], Sailaja Urpayil[3,4] and Mohamed Shahin Thayyil[1]

1 Department of Physics, University of Calicut, Malappuram, India

2 Department of Physics, Kottakkal Farook Arts and Science College, Kottakkal, Kerala, India

3 Department of Physics, M E S Keveeyam College, Valanchery, Kerala, India

4 Department of Physics, MES Ponnani College, Ponnani, Malappuram, Kerala, India

*Address all correspondence to: safnahussain2@gmail.com

References

[1] Lewars, E., 2004. Computational Chemistry; Introduction to the Theory and Applications of Molecular and Quantum Mechanics, KLUWER ACADEMIC PUBLISHERS

[2] Masoud Soroush, 2018, Computational Quantum Chemistry; First Edition, Elsevier

[3] G. Ramachandran, S. Muthu, J. Uma Maheswari, Density functional theory and Ab initio studies of vibrational spectroscopic (FT-IR, FT-Raman and UV) first order hyperpolarizabilities, NBO, HOMO-LUMO and TD-DFT analysis of the 1,2-Dihydropyrazolo (4,3-E) Pyrimidin-4-one, Solid State Sci. 16 (2013) 45-5

[4] Errol G. Lewars, 2011, Computational Chemistry Introduction to the Theory and Applications of Molecular and Quantum Mechanics; Second Edition, Springer Dordrecht Heidelberg London New York

[5] K.P Safna Hussan, M.Shahin Thayyil, V.K. Rajan, K. Muraleedharan, DFT studies on global parameters, antioxidant mechanism and molecular docking of amlodipine besylate, Comput. Biol. Chem. 80 (2019) 46-53. doi:10.1016/j.compbiolchem.2019.03.006

[6] David C. Young, 2001, COMPUTATIONAL CHEMISTRY A Practical Guide for Applying Techniques to Real-World Problems; first ed,A JOHN WILEY & SONS, INC., PUBLICATION

[7] Introduction to Gaussian: Theory and Practice; gaussian Inc 2015. Chennai India

[8] British National Formulary, 2008, BMJ Group and RPS Publishing

[9] 1998-2020 International Foundation for Gastrointestinal Disorders, Inc. (IFFGD)

[10] E.E. Bolton, Y. Wang, P.A. Thiessen, S.H. Bryant, Integrated Platform of Small Molecules and Biological Activities, in: R.A.W. and D.C.S.B.T.-A.R. in C. Chemistry (Ed.), Elsevier, 2008: pp. 217-241.

[11] N.M. O'Boyle, M. Banck, C.A. James, C. Morley, T. Vandermeersch, G.R. Hutchison, Open Babel: An open chemical toolbox. ., J. Chem. Informatics. 3 (2011) 33

[12] K.P. Safna Hussan, M. Shahin Thayyil, Vijisha K. Rajan, K. Muraleedharan 2017 Experimental and density functional theory studies on benzalkonium ibuprofenate, a double active pharmaceutical ingredient Computational Biology and Chemistry 72(2018) 113-121

[13] Vijisha K. Rajan, K. Muraleedharan., 2017. A computational investigation on the structure, global parameters and antioxidant capacity of a polyphenol, Gallic acid. Food Chem. 220, 93-99

[14] R. Meenakshi, Spectral investigations, DFT based global reactivity descriptors, Inhibition efficiency and analysis of 5-chloro-2-nitroanisole as π-spacer with donor-acceptor variations effect for DSSCs performance, J. Mol. Struct. 1127 (2017) 694-707

[15] Di Zhou, An Introduction of Density Functional Theory and its Application; lecture

[16] Silverstein, R.M., Bassler, G.C., Morrill, T.C., 1991. Spectrometric identification of organic compounds, fifth ed. John Wiley & Sons, Singapore

[17] T. Rajamani, S. Muthu, Electronic absorption, vibrational spectra, non-linear optical properties, NBO analysis and thermodynamic properties of 9-[(2-hydroxyethoxy) methyl] guanine

molecule by density functional method, Solid State Sci. 16 (2013) 90-101

[18] G. Ramachandran, S. Muthu, J. Uma Maheswari, Density functional theory and Ab initio studies of vibrational spectroscopic (FT-IR, FT-Raman and UV) first order hyperpolarizabilities, NBO, HOMO-LUMO and TD-DFT analysis of the 1,2-Dihydropyrazolo (4,3-E) Pyrimidin-4-one, Solid State Sci. 16 (2013) 45-52.

[19] Christopher J. Cramer, 2004, Essentials of Computational Chemistry Theories and Models; Second Edition, John Wiley & Sons Ltd

[20] K.G. Sangeetha, K.K. Aravindakshan, K.P. Safna Hussan, Insight into the theoretical and experimental studies of 1-phenyl-3-methyl-4-benzoyl-5-pyrazolone N (4)-methyl- N (4)- phenylthiosemicarbazone - A potential NLO material, J. Mol. Struct. 1150 (2017) 135-145. doi:10.1016/j.molstruc.2017.08.078

[21] U. Sailaja, M. Shahin Thayyil , N.S. Krishna Kumar, G. Govindaraj , K.L. Ngai, Molecular mobility in the super cooled and glassy states of Nizatidine and Perphenazine. European Journal of Pharmaceutical Sciences 99 (2017) 147-151.

[22] K.P. Safna Hussan, M. Shahin Thayyil, S.K. Deshpande, T.V. Jinitha, V.K. Rajan, K.L. Ngai, Synthesis and molecular dynamics of double active pharmaceutical ingredient-benzalkonium ibuprofenate, J. Mol. Liq. 223 (2016) 1333-1339. doi:10.1016/j.molliq.2016.09.054.